MW00561083

THE EASY HEART HEALTHY COOKBOOK FOR SLOW COOKERS

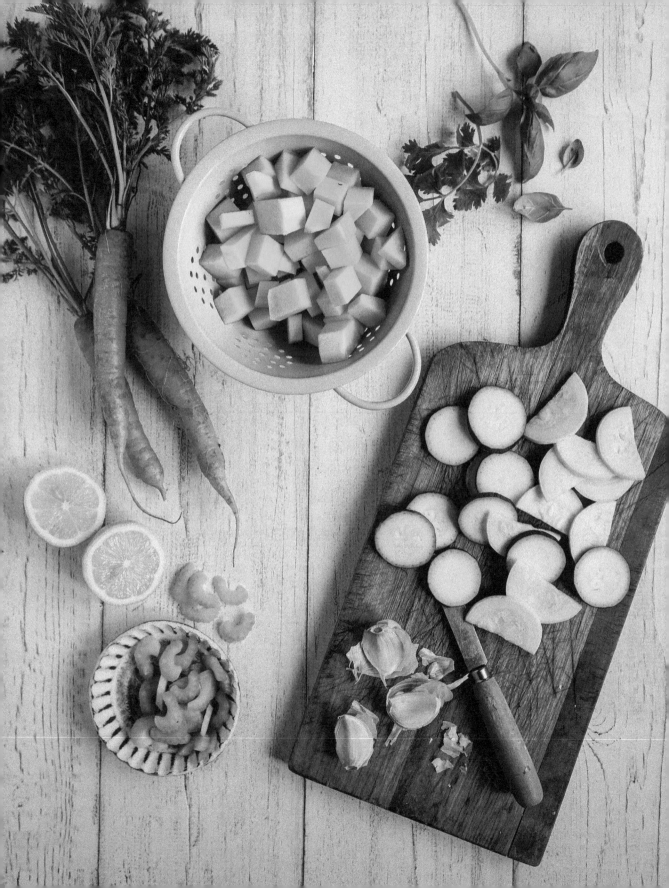

THE EASY
Heart Healthy
Cookbook
FOR SLOW COOKERS

130 Prep-and-Go Low-Sodium Recipes

Nicole R. Morrissey **MS, RD, CDE**

PHOTOGRAPHY BY HÉLÈNE DUJARDIN

ROCKRIDGE PRESS

Copyright © 2018 by Nicole R. Morrissey

No part of this publication may be reproduced, stored in a retrieval system, or transmitted in any form or by any means, electronic, mechanical, photocopying, recording, scanning, or otherwise, except as permitted under Sections 107 or 108 of the 1976 United States Copyright Act, without the prior written permission of the Publisher. Requests to the Publisher for permission should be addressed to the Permissions Department, Rockridge Press, 6005 Shellmound Street, Suite 175, Emeryville, CA 94608.

Limit of Liability/Disclaimer of Warranty: The Publisher and the author make no representations or warranties with respect to the accuracy or completeness of the contents of this work and specifically disclaim all warranties, including without limitation warranties of fitness for a particular purpose. No warranty may be created or extended by sales or promotional materials. The advice and strategies contained herein may not be suitable for every situation. This work is sold with the understanding that the Publisher is not engaged in rendering medical, legal, or other professional advice or services. If professional assistance is required, the services of a competent professional person should be sought. Neither the Publisher nor the author shall be liable for damages arising herefrom. The fact that an individual, organization, or website is referred to in this work as a citation and/or potential source of further information does not mean that the author or the Publisher endorses the information the individual, organization, or website may provide or recommendations they/it may make. Further, readers should be aware that Internet websites listed in this work may have changed or disappeared between when this work was written and when it is read.

For general information on our other products and services or to obtain technical support, please contact our Customer Care Department within the United States at (866) 744-2665, or outside the United States at (510) 253-0500.

Rockridge Press publishes its books in a variety of electronic and print formats. Some content that appears in print may not be available in electronic books, and vice versa.

TRADEMARKS: Rockridge Press and the Rockridge Press logo are trademarks or registered trademarks of Callisto Media Inc. and/or its affiliates, in the United States and other countries, and may not be used without written permission. All other trademarks are the property of their respective owners. Rockridge Press is not associated with any product or vendor mentioned in this book.

Photorgraphy @ Hélène Dujardin, 2018; Food styling by Tami Hardeman

ISBN: Print 978-1-64152-086-7 | eBook 978-1-64152-087-4

To my loving husband, who always
offers up the unadulterated truth
in all things. Including food.

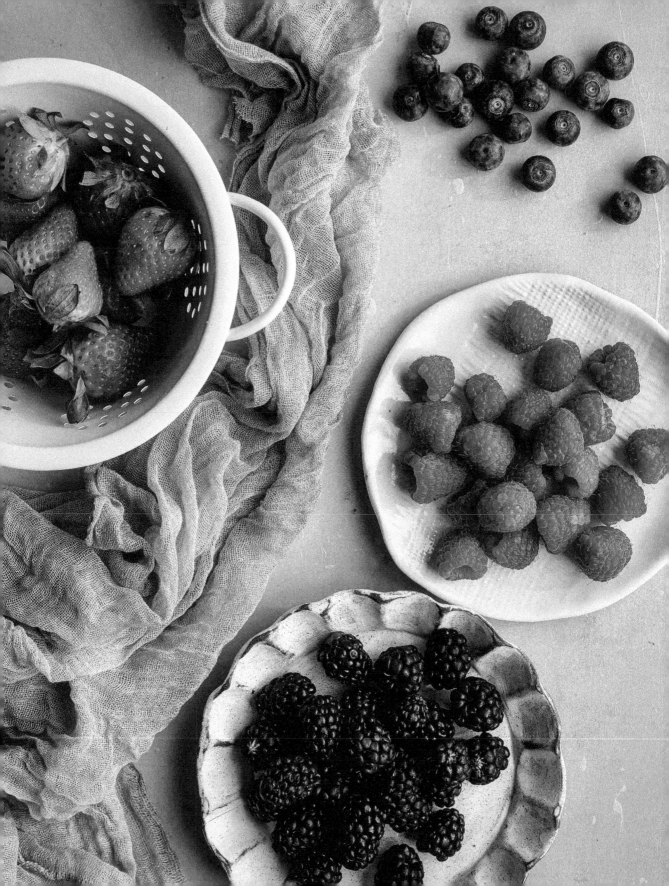

CONTENTS

INTRODUCTION

We all seem to find ourselves short on time. Of all the tasks that are necessary to get us from day to day, cooking is one that quickly falls by the wayside. We can easily opt for convenience foods and meals away from home that can lead to a diet that isn't healthy for our hearts.

According to the Centers for Disease Control and Prevention, heart disease is the leading cause of death in the United States, accounting for more than 50 percent of people's deaths in 2015. Modifiable risk factors for heart disease include diet, body weight, physical activity, diabetes, and alcohol intake. Eating a heart-healthy diet can play a huge role in weight loss, if needed, and in maintaining or regaining heart health.

As a Registered Dietitian, I have the privilege of helping people improve their lives through changes to their diet. I'll be the first to admit that eating a heart-healthy diet can be challenging within the demands of our busy lives. I'll also be the first to tell you it's entirely possible to do so, even when you're short on time or inexperienced in the kitchen. The slow cooker can be a lifesaver (*pun intended!*) when it comes to getting a meal on the table that can best support your heart-healthy lifestyle.

When I got married in 2009, my cooking experience was limited to what I had used to survive through college—a jar of marinara heated on the stove top with a ton of vegetables thrown in, served over a bed of whole-wheat pasta. Although my passion for nutrition had been set in motion, it was those early days of marriage that developed my love for cooking. Having the knowledge and skills to put a balanced, heart-healthy meal on the table for my husband and myself was important to me. I had forever struggled with my weight and knew my family had a long history of heart disease, so eating a heart-healthy diet that limited sodium and saturated fat while including generous amounts of fiber was my priority. Beyond the healthiness of the meal, I also knew I had to create food that tasted *amazing*. If your food is uninspiring and tasteless, your heart-healthy efforts will be short-lived.

A slow cooker is the ideal appliance for preparing heart-healthy food. The low-and-slow cooking method promotes taste and texture without added fat or salt. When my clients start using their slow cookers to prepare simple recipes,

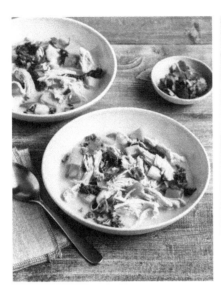
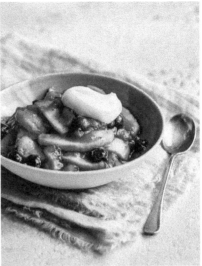

they quickly realize how easy improving their diet can be. That's the best part of being a dietitian—helping people experience that lightbulb moment when they recognize that creating easy meals at home can keep them healthy and still allow them to enjoy their meals.

Today, I also have little mouths to feed. Two of them! Motherhood combined with a full-time job can leave me desperately short on time. I've become more reliant than ever on my slow cooker, and in recent years have perfected the art of simple prep-and-go meals that are perfect for a heart-healthy lifestyle.

The recipes in this book were designed with the ease of the slow cooker in mind. You won't find mandatory precooking requirements in here; just prep everything and throw it in the slow cooker. And most main dishes cook for 8 hours, ensuring that you can go to work and come home to dinner. It's my hope that these recipes will help you maintain your diet and health, and live your best life.

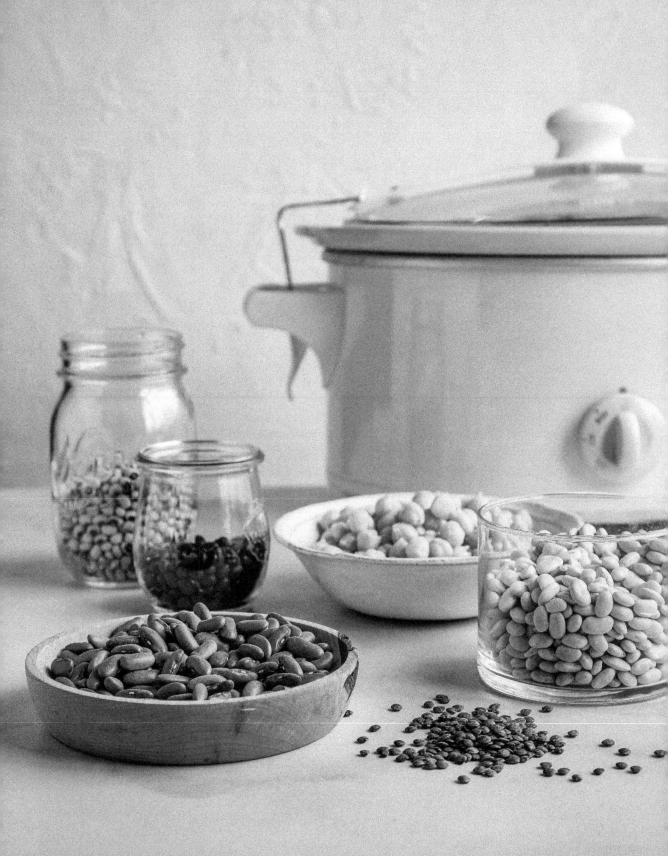

1

Slow Cook for Heart Health

Slow cooking is practical, easy, and delicious. If you've ever used a slow cooker, I know I don't have much convincing to do. Whether you are a slow cooker novice or already a slow cooker convert, the recipes and tips in this book will help you use this great tool to prepare heart-healthy meals.

EATING FOR HEART HEALTH

When we give consideration to not just eating but also eating healthily, we are often left with more questions than answers. What's a heart-healthy diet, anyway? What should we eat to combat or prevent heart disease?

It's important to understand that what's healthy for one individual may not be healthy for someone else. Nutrition is *not* a one-size-fits-all science, so we must determine where nutrition and heart health intersect. To do that, we need to consider three major components to the diet: sodium, fat, and fiber. Let's break this down a bit.

SODIUM: High blood pressure is one of the major risk factors for heart disease, but limiting the sodium in your diet can help stabilize blood pressure. Sodium is responsible for fluid balance in the body, and excess sodium pulls water into the blood vessels. This uptick in blood volume results in the body needing to pump more blood and, as a result, the pressure within the blood vessels increases. Over time, this increased pressure can cause harm to the vessel walls and contribute to the buildup of plaque that can impede blood flow. A low-sodium diet can reduce your risk of headaches and heart attacks.

FAT: Adhering to a diet low in saturated and trans fats promotes healthy blood cholesterol levels. With excess saturated fat, low-density lipoprotein (LDL) cholesterol (the bad stuff) rises. Worse yet, trans fats cause LDL cholesterol to rise and cardio-protective high-density lipoprotein (HDL) cholesterol (the good stuff) to decrease. Incorporating monounsaturated and polyunsaturated fats can help reduce LDL cholesterol levels, thus reducing the risk of heart disease and stroke. Omega-3 fatty acids—found in fish, canola oil, walnuts, and flaxseed—are essential to good health and not produced by the body, so we must rely on food to obtain them.

FIBER: Eating a diet high in fiber helps reduce both blood pressure and LDL cholesterol levels. Fiber remains undigested and helps promote a healthy gut biome while providing satiety—an incredibly helpful component of a successful meal plan. Foods that contain 5 or more grams of dietary fiber in a single serving can be considered high-fiber foods. These foods are often also rich in B vitamins, folate, iron, and magnesium.

SODIUM

Sodium, commonly referred to as salt, is in virtually everything we eat. And we need it—just not too much of it. Most of us are aware that we should go easy on the salt shaker, or eliminate it altogether, but the salt that's found in prepared and prepackaged foods provides, by and large, the bulk of the sodium we consume—about 75 percent. Even "reduced-sodium" foods can be quite high in sodium.

The nutrition facts label is the best place to find the total sodium content in the packaged foods we eat. Sodium is often listed as any number of sodium-containing ingredients, such as monosodium glutamate, sodium nitrate, or sodium citrate to name just a few. Be watchful of the serving size indicated on the label and adjust the amount used accordingly.

So, how much is too much? This is often different for each person, but a good place to start is a range of 1,500 to 2,300 milligrams a day. One thing to remember: When you get used to looking at individual ingredient labels, the sodium content for entire prepared meals can sometimes seem alarmingly high. I've limited the sodium for each recipe to no more than 700 milligrams *per serving*. These meals can also be balanced out with lower-sodium meals and snacks that include little or no sodium, such as fresh fruits and vegetables. For reference, foods that have less than 140 milligrams per serving can be considered low-sodium items, and foods that contain less than 5 milligrams per serving can be considered sodium-free.

In general, we eat too much sodium. If you're older than 50, are African American, or have hypertension, chronic kidney disease, diabetes, or heart failure, you are in a high-risk category and should closely evaluate your intake of sodium. If you're not sure how much salt you consume each day, start by totaling your intake based on nutrition labels. Increasing the number of potassium-rich foods in your diet can help you decrease your sodium intake, help lower blood pressure, and help the heart muscles function optimally. I've included the use of some salt substitutes, such as Mrs. Dash, in the recipes. Salt substitutes can be found in nearly every grocery store and can help enhance flavor without adding unwanted sodium.

FAT

Limiting our saturated fat and trans fat intake is integral to heart health. Try to limit saturated fat to no more than 13 grams a day, or about 5 to 6 percent of calories. Saturated fat is the primary diet-related driver for an elevated LDL cholesterol level. Choosing lean meats and low-fat or fat-free dairy, and incorporating vegetarian options are all great ways to reduce saturated fat in the diet. Along those same lines, choosing reduced-fat ingredients and condiments can drastically reduce the amount of saturated fat you eat.

Trans fats can be found in many prepared foods in the form of partially hydrogenated oils. Checking the ingredient list for partially hydrogenated oil of any kind is crucial to identifying trans fat because amounts less than 0.5 gram per serving are not required to be listed on the nutrition facts label. Although some animal products contain small amounts of naturally occurring trans fat, the vast majority of trans fat in our diet is from processed foods, such as doughnuts, cakes, biscuits, frozen pizza, cookies, crackers, and margarine.

A helpful trick is to use liquid oils instead of solid fats when possible. Liquid oils (other than tropical oils, such as room-temperature palm and coconut oils) are high in heart-healthy monounsaturated and polyunsaturated fats. Other sources of healthy unsaturated fats include nuts and nut butters, seeds, fish, avocado, and olives. But be mindful of the sodium content in some of these foods.

FIBER

A professor of mine once explained dietary fiber as the janitors of the body. Soluble fiber is especially helpful in improving cholesterol levels and optimizing heart health. Found in whole grains, legumes, fruits, and vegetables, soluble fiber should be abundant in the diet. Dietary fiber includes both soluble and insoluble fiber, and adults should aim for at least 25 to 30 grams each day.

THE BENEFITS OF SLOW COOKING

Here are seven ways slow cooking promotes heart health:

1. It is a great way to make at least half of your grains whole grains and incorporate more fiber into your diet. Steel-cut oats, bulgur, brown rice, barley, and quinoa are perfect in the slow cooker—they take longer to cook than the more processed options, so plugging in the slow cooker and walking away is a time-saving, no-fuss option.

2. Leaner meats that are low in saturated fat are best prepared using moist heat, which can be achieved with a low-and-slow cooking approach. The slow cooker tenderizes the collagen in the meat, creating juicy proteins without all the fat. Your meat will be tender and flavorful.

3. The slow cooker is ideal for soups and stews packed with beans, vegetables, and lean meat. Get creative with various spices and ingredients to add flavor in lieu of salt. This helps drastically reduce the amount of sodium that can be found in canned and prepared soups.

4. Breakfast, truly the most important meal of the day, is a cinch in a slow cooker! Don't let breakfast go uneaten—preparing breakfast as you sleep is a total time-saver. Plus, you'll likely have leftovers to enjoy throughout the week.

More Time to Get Active

Undeniably, diet plays a significant role in maintaining and improving heart health … but so does *exercise*. Yes, it can be a challenge to carve out that time for exercise in our busy lives, but doing so is rewarding for your mind, body, and heart. I love to say, "You never regret a workout!" because it's so very true. It can be hard to get started, but it's doubly rewarding to have done it on the days when it seemed the most difficult.

Using a slow cooker frees up the time you would have spent in the kitchen preparing meals so you can get outside and be active, hit the gym, or find another way to get moving. Slow cooking helps remove excuses and can help improve and maintain health.

One way to be sure your exercise routine is not overlooked is to be consistent about the time of day and days of the week you exercise. Making a plan and sticking to it dissuades us from putting off important activities, especially those we want to develop into habits. Schedule slow cooker meals for the days you plan to exercise—spend the time you'd normally devote to meal preparation to exercise while your meal is slowly cooking.

Most important, find an exercise you enjoy! Start slow and don't overdo it. You don't want to be discouraged by unrealistic goals … and don't want to injure yourself, either. Try something new. If you don't enjoy what you're doing—or eating—you won't adhere to any changes in the long term. Slow cooking can help you get creative and get moving, all without sacrificing the home-cooked meals that can help you achieve your best heart health.

5. You can have dinner piping hot and ready to eat the minute you walk in the door. This eliminates the temptation of dining out or picking up takeout. The slow cooker is a foolproof plan for incorporating heart-healthy meals into even the busiest times.

6. Flavors are optimally distributed throughout the dish thanks to the extended cooking times. Be sure not to overfill your slow cooker—it should never be more than two-thirds full. Allowing air circulation around the food is an important piece of the slow-cooking process. You can create big flavors without too much salt or fat.

7. The slow cooker turns fiber-rich lentils, peas, and beans into little nuggets of flavor. These foods take a considerable amount of time to cook on the stove top so they're perfect to whip up in the slow cooker, cooking to perfection with minimal effort.

A HEART-HEALTHY KITCHEN

Fat and salt play a role in the taste and texture of prepared meals—and there's no denying that we all want to eat flavorful meals. Uniquely, slow cooking offers both the taste and texture benefits of salty, high-fat meal preparation while ditching the excess fats and sodium-packed ingredients. The low-and-slow cooking method maximizes flavors and textures while keeping meals simple, tasty, *and* heart healthy without excessive fat and sodium. Lean meats that are quickly made into dry, tough bricks on the stove top, will instead braise into tender and juicy meals . . . while legumes and soups attain their finest taste with far less effort and time on your part. Setting up your pantry for slow cooking is a sure way to eat well, save time, and achieve a more healthy heart. This section will provide a rundown on superfoods that are great for both the slow cooker and for your heart health, as well as guidelines on how to make the most out of your slow cooker.

SLOW COOKER SUPERFOODS

Keep your pantry packed with slow-cooking essentials. Having these ingredients on hand will help eliminate the daily question *"What are we going to eat?"* These slow cooker superfoods promote heart health and are delicious when slow cooked.

Pantry Essentials

Buy nonperishables when they're on sale. Not only will you keep your kitchen stocked, you'll also save money.

BEANS. Beans are high in protein and offer 7 grams of fiber in a ½-cup serving! Black beans are flavonoid-rich, helping the arteries of your heart stay healthy.

LENTILS. Going meat-free is a great way to both increase fiber and slash saturated fat intake. A ½ cup serving of lentils also offers half your daily folate needs and a host of B vitamins.

QUINOA. With all 20 amino acids, quinoa is a true gem—or should I say seed? High in both fiber and protein, it is unique in its protein-to-carbohydrate ratio, making it more balanced than grains.

STEEL-CUT OATS. Thanks to their hearty nature, steel-cut oats are often bypassed for more processed old-fashioned or quick oats. But steel-cut oats make the perfect slow cooker breakfast. With extreme staying power, they are a good source of iron and a slow cooker superfood.

SWEET POTATOES. A richer source of fiber than white potatoes, sweet potatoes also offer higher concentrations of most nutrients while becoming tender and sweet in the slow cooker.

BARLEY. A specific fiber in barley, beta-glucan, goes to work to lower cholesterol in the body making it a heart-healthy grain that holds up great in slow cooking.

CANNED TOMATOES. Canning tomatoes at their peak ripeness ensures the best taste and nutrition. Available in no-salt-added varieties, canned tomatoes are high in lycopene, which has been linked with a decreased risk of heart attack.

POTATOES. Sweet potatoes get a lot of well-deserved press, but it's the plain old spud that offers powerful blood pressure–lowering potassium. Despite their questionable reputation, it's what goes *on* or in the potato that can diminish its superfood status rather than the potato itself.

PEANUT BUTTER. High in arginine—an amino acid that helps keep blood vessels healthy—and abundant in heart-healthy unsaturated fat, peanut butter turns ooey and gooey in the slow cooker. A little bit goes a long way and that creamy, rich flavor can turn a dessert (or breakfast!) into a true superfood treat.

EXTRA-VIRGIN OLIVE OIL AND OLIVE OIL-BASED NONSTICK COOKING SPRAY. The body needs fat, but choosing wholesome, heart-healthy sources of fat is key. High in monounsaturated fat and extensively researched for its positive effect on heart health, extra-virgin olive oil is arguably the best oil to incorporate into a heart-healthy diet.

Refrigerator Essentials

Keep your refrigerator full of slow cooker essentials. It helps keep no-fuss, heart-healthy meals on the menu during your busy week.

MINCED GARLIC. Yes, fresh garlic has better flavor . . . but the convenience of having garlic ready to throw into the slow cooker can be a very helpful timesaver. And the anti-oxidant allicin found in garlic can be helpful in regulating blood pressure.

BONELESS, SKINLESS CHICKEN BREASTS. A blank slate for flavor and extremely low in saturated fat, chicken breasts are ideal for the slow cooker and can morph into any number of delicious meals, from soups to stews to mains.

SALSA. Salsas are a sneaky and flavorful way to get vegetables into a meal. Look for salsas that are lower in sodium. If you like a little spice, buy medium or hot salsa—a little bit goes a long way while keeping the sodium in check.

LOW-FAT OR FAT-FREE PLAIN GREEK YOGURT. With double the amount of protein than traditional yogurt, Greek yogurt adds a thick and creamy texture to slow cooker meals. Always turn off the slow cooker and stir the yogurt in just before serving to avoid separation.

LOW-FAT CHEESE. There's no denying a little bit of cheese can really make a meal special. Opt for low-fat varieties that offer both great taste and meltability but without all the added fat.

SQUEEZE-TUBE HERBS. Rather than buying fresh herbs by the bunch or in a big package—which is often more than you need—buy prepared herbs to save time and money and get flavor that is much fresher than that of dried herbs. It's a bonus that they're made without added salt and keep for several months in the refrigerator.

NO-SALT-ADDED BROTHS. The slow cooker relies on liquid ingredients for preparing most recipes and these broths are commonplace now in most grocery stores. Have them on hand for when you aren't able to make your own. They add big flavor with less sodium.

EGGS. With 6 to 7 grams of protein and a mere 70 calories, eggs are nutrient-dense and versatile. Low in saturated fat, eggs are a powerful disease-fighting food that is naturally low in sodium. Although eggs were previously shunned for their cholesterol content, the latest research disputes that their cholesterol is harmful to heart health.

5 Foods You Should NOT Slow Cook

All right, the slow cooker is a wonderful tool that can help support efforts to lead a heart-healthy lifestyle . . . but it's not ideal for preparing all foods. There are a select few foods that you should not slow cook. Their delicate texture or intolerance to prolonged heat makes these foods appropriate for traditional stove top or oven preparations.

Fish. Though incredibly important to a heart-healthy diet, fish is simply not a food to slow cook. It cannot hold its shape and withstand the prolonged cooking time.

Seafood. Scallops, oysters, shrimp, lobster, and crab all cook in a matter of minutes and therefore turn rubbery in a slow cooker. Save time and prepare using the stove top or oven.

Delicate fresh vegetables. Most vegetables hold up well in the slow cooker, but asparagus, eggplant, tomatoes, and zucchini should be prepared using another cooking method.

Delicate fresh fruits. Many fruits are suitable for the slow cooker, but bananas, kiwi, citrus, and melon are better when eaten raw or cooked with alternate techniques.

Couscous. Even heartier whole-wheat couscous can't hold up in a slow cooker. Choose almost any other grain to swap into your recipe: barley, millet, teff, farro, kamut, and so forth.

FLAXSEED. Be sure to store ground flaxseed in the refrigerator. Flaxseed, which is high in omega-3 fatty acids, can be incorporated into many recipes, like oatmeal and casseroles.

CURRY PASTE. One little jar of green or red curry paste can create beautiful Asian flavors in many of your slow cooker meals. Store the jar in the refrigerator after opening. A little bit goes a long way and a tablespoon of curry paste has about half the amount of sodium as a tablespoon of reduced-sodium soy sauce.

KNOW YOUR SLOW COOKER

A 6-quart slow cooker is the most standard size, making recipes that serve 6 to 8 people on average, so a 6-quart slow cooker was used for the recipes in this book unless otherwise specified. To prepare truly delicious meals, be sure your slow cooker is not too big or too small. You do not want to overfill or underfill your slow cooker. To get the best results, your slow cooker should be roughly half to two-thirds full. If your slow cooker is underfilled, plan to adjust the cooking time down by 1 to 2 hours. Similarly, adjust the cooking time up by 1 to 2 hours for a slow cooker that is fuller. I find that the low setting is often best when it comes to allowing flavors to develop, soups to thicken, and meats to become fork-tender, but each recipe will note the cooking time on high and low, where possible, so the cooking time can be adapted to fit your schedule.

The shape of your slow cooker—round or oval—has more to do with what you intend to make than its functionality. Although soups and stews can be prepared in any shaped slow cooker, a whole chicken often fits best in an oval. When you are purchasing a slow cooker, consider the ease with which you can clean it by hand or fit it into the dishwasher. I highly recommend a slow cooker with a removable insert for ease of cleaning, as well as for prepping meals ahead of time and storing them in the refrigerator for later slow cooking. If your slow cooker doesn't have a removable insert, you can purchase liners at the grocery store; they're in the aisle with the plastic wrap and aluminum foil. Slow cooker liners are a completely optional way to make cleanup easier. Some people swear by them, others can take them or leave them.

Slow cookers can vary in their features, including the type of lid, timer, and heat settings. A snug-fitting lid ensures heat stays captured in the slow cooker. Some slow cookers are even built with clasps to secure the lid to the base, ensuring a tight seal and disaster-free transport should you take your slow cooker meal away from home. Additionally, a glass lid allows you a sneak peek at the contents without lifting the lid and disrupting the slow-cooking process. A timer can be a helpful feature if there may be a lag between the end of cooking and your arrival home. Using the timer feature stops the cooking process to prevent overcooking. Finally, the heat settings on slow cookers may

Slow Cooker Dos and Don'ts

DOS

1. Use the right-sized slow cooker for best results.
2. Use the timer to prevent overcooking and accommodate your schedule.
3. Use liners for easy cleanup.
4. Trim meat before slow cooking to cut saturated fat.
5. Choose the right foods—not all foods are suitable for the slow cooker.

DON'TS

1. Stir. It's tempting to stir the contents of the slow cooker during the cooking process, but you should allow the slow cooker to do the work.
2. Lift the lid. Heat escapes when you lift the lid, which disrupts the cooking and adds additional cook time (about 20 minutes for every peek).
3. Cook too long. To prevent dry or tough results, don't extend cook times, if possible.
4. Use frozen foods. Using frozen foods keeps the slow cooker contents in the "danger zone" between 40°F and 140°F for unsafe lengths of time. Thaw frozen foods before adding to the slow cooker.
5. Add dairy too soon. Add dairy at the end of cooking to prevent separation and curdling.

vary. While almost every slow cooker comes equipped with high and low settings, many offer features such as "keep warm" or "buffet" to keep foods heated versus continuing to cook. But even a very basic slow cooker should do the trick for the recipes in this book. I focused my efforts here on truly no-fuss meals that allow you to prep and go without fancy settings or additional stove top steps, whenever possible.

ABOUT THE RECIPES

My goal in this book is to provide you with recipes that are simple, delicious, and heart-healthy. Expect to see recipes that are truly prep-and-go meals that don't require precooking, hard-to-find ingredients, or anything that's not doable as a weeknight meal. Most recipes cook for eight hours, so you can throw everything in the slow cooker, go about your day, and come home to dinner. The prep time listed is a guesstimate. It takes into account the time needed to gather ingredients and tools and to get everything into the slow cooker and ready to turn on. I know you're busy and that eating well for your heart has to be something you can maintain and enjoy—forever.

You'll also see several labels throughout the cookbook, including:

ALLERGY-FREE—none of the top eight allergens: wheat, eggs, milk, fish, shellfish, soy, peanuts, or tree nuts

DAIRY-FREE—free of milk, yogurt, cheese, and other dairy-containing ingredients

GLUTEN-FREE—no gluten (wheat, barley, rye)

NUT-FREE—no tree nuts or peanuts

VEGAN—no meat, dairy, or animal products

VEGETARIAN—no meat or meat products

To take even better advantage of the time-saving aspects of slow cooking, try prepping food ahead of time. Vegetables can be chopped, meat can be trimmed, and spices can be measured. Use convenience foods like prechopped onion, celery, and winter squash that are available in most grocery store produce departments. Feel free to substitute in different ingredients to suit your preferences—just be sure to limit or avoid added salt and high-sodium condiments. Instead, use herbs to enhance flavor.

Each recipe in the book includes a full panel of nutrition facts (based on the list of ingredients for each recipe) so you not only know what's in the food you're eating, but you can also make the best decisions for your health. When alternate ingredients are listed in the ingredients list (e.g., when you have a choice of low-fat, fat-free, or plant-based milk), the nutritional information is based on the first ingredient listed. And many recipes include suggestions for ways *to serve* the recipe, but those ingredients or preparations are not included in the nutritional information.

Now all that's left is to enjoy the robust flavors, tender textures, and fragrant delights that will fill your home with great aromas and your stomach with delicious food while keeping your heart healthy and strong!

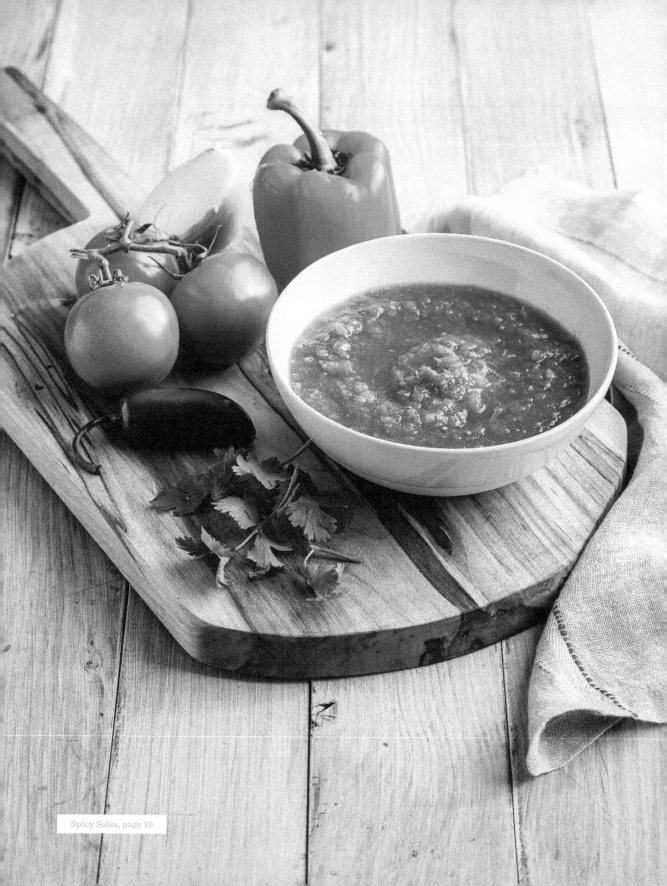

Spicy Salsa, page 19

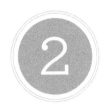

Staples

RUSTIC MARINARA SAUCE

Prep time: 5 minutes / Cook time: 7 to 8 hours on low

This classic Italian marinara sauce has the best flavor because it is cooked in the slow cooker using fresh tomatoes, herbs, and vegetables, allowing the ingredients to develop and deepen. It's perfect for topping whole-grain pasta, pizza, spiralized vegetables, or your favorite meats, and it can be used as is or you can add other favorite ingredients, like mushrooms and spinach. Freeze in 1- to 2-cup portions so it's always convenient to have on hand.

Makes about 12 cups

6 pounds Roma
  tomatoes, chopped

1 (6-ounce) can tomato paste

6 garlic cloves, minced

1 large onion, finely chopped

1 medium red bell
  pepper, chopped

1 medium carrot, shredded

2 teaspoons dried basil

1 teaspoon dried oregano

½ teaspoon dried thyme

½ teaspoon dried marjoram

½ teaspoon crushed red
  pepper flakes (optional)

1. Combine all the ingredients in a 6-quart slow cooker. Cover and cook on low for 7 to 8 hours.

2. If desired, use an immersion blender after cooking to crush the tomatoes to desired consistency.

3. Use immediately or freeze in 1- to 2-cup portions in airtight containers for up to 4 months.

Per Serving (1 cup): Calories: 71; Total Fat: 0g; Saturated Fat: 0g; Trans Fat: 0g; Polyunsaturated Fat: 0g; Monounsaturated Fat: 0g; Cholesterol: 0g; Sodium: 137mg; Carbohydrates: 16g; Fiber: 4g; Sugars: 9g; Protein: 3g

NUTRITIONAL HIGHLIGHT: An excellent source of vitamin C, potassium, and fiber, tomatoes are high in the phytonutrient lycopene, which works with other nutrients for disease prevention, including preventing cardiovascular disease. Cooking actually increases the health benefits as it makes their phytonutrients more available.

ITALIAN BOLOGNESE SAUCE

Prep time: 15 minutes / Cook time: 7 to 8 hours on low

This Bolognese sauce uses fresh tomatoes and is slow cooked for hours to give it that rich, delicious flavor. Serve this sauce over vegetable noodles or whole-grain pasta, or in your favorite lasagna recipe. It's also perfect for freezing. Using honey and red wine is entirely optional, but they add a nice touch of flavor; they are not included in the nutritional analysis.

Makes 8 cups

1 tablespoon extra-virgin olive oil (optional)

1 pound 93% lean ground beef

1 medium onion, roughly chopped

4 garlic cloves, minced

5 to 6 pounds tomatoes, seeded and chopped

1 medium carrot, roughly chopped

1 dried bay leaf

1 teaspoon dried oregano

1 teaspoon dried basil

¼ cup tomato paste

Freshly ground black pepper

Honey (optional)

¼ cup red wine (optional)

1. Optional step: In a large skillet, heat the oil over medium-high heat. Add the ground beef, onion, and garlic. Cover and cook stirring frequently until beef is browned, 7 to 10 minutes. Drain any excess fat and liquid from the beef.

2. Combine the beef, onion, garlic, tomatoes, carrot, bay leaf, oregano, basil, tomato paste, black pepper, honey (if using), and wine (if using) in a 6-quart slow cooker. Stir to combine. Cover and cook on low for 7 to 8 hours or until the sauce is thickened.

3. Remove and discard the bay leaf.

4. Serve warm or freeze in 1- to 2-cup portions in airtight containers for up to 3 months.

Per Serving (1 cup): Calories: 182; Total Fat: 6g; Saturated Fat: 2g; Trans Fat: 0g; Polyunsaturated Fat: 1g; Monounsaturated Fat: 2g; Cholesterol: 32mg; Sodium: 131mg; Carbohydrates: 17g; Fiber: 5g; Sugars: 11g; Protein: 16g

VARIATION TIP: You can replace the ground beef with ground white meat turkey or ground pork depending on your tastes. You could also add 1 cup of chopped button mushrooms to enhance the flavor and boost the fiber content.

CREAMY VEGAN ALFREDO SAUCE

Prep time: 5 minutes / Cook time: 7 to 8 hours on low or 3 to 4 hours on high

This vegan Alfredo sauce uses heart-healthy cashews in place of heavy cream, butter, and cheese. The liquid from the broth and water will soak and soften the cashews, making them easy to blend at the end of cooking with an immersion blender. Serve with vegetable noodles or whole-grain pasta, or as a topping for baked potatoes.

Makes about 4 cups

3 cups Savory Vegetable Broth (page 24) or low-sodium vegetable broth

1 cup raw cashews

1 cup water

½ cup unsweetened soymilk

½ cup nutritional yeast

1 teaspoon dried mustard

2 garlic cloves, minced

Juice of ½ lemon

Pinch salt

1. Combine all the ingredients in a 6-quart slow cooker and stir well. Cover and cook on low for 7 to 8 hours, until the cashews are softened.

2. Purée the sauce until smooth using an immersion blender.

3. Serve warm.

Per Serving (½ cup): Calories: 133; Total Fat: 9g; Saturated Fat: 1g; Trans Fat: 0g; Polyunsaturated Fat: 0g; Monounsaturated Fat: 0g; Cholesterol: 0mg; Sodium: 79mg; Carbohydrates: 10g; Fiber: 2g; Sugars: 2g; Protein: 8g

SUBSTITUTION TIP: Nutritional yeast is grown on molasses or in a similar habitat and is known for its tangy, cheesy flavor. It is a rich source of B vitamins and a complete plant-based protein. Found in the health-food section of most grocery stores or in the baking aisle, you can easily swap it for Parmesan cheese—just note that the sauce will no longer be vegan if you use the cheese.

SPICY SALSA

Prep time: 10 minutes / Cook time: 7 to 8 hours on low

This restaurant-style garden salsa has so many delicious and fresh ingredients and uses up all of those summer garden tomatoes. What's better than homemade salsa to serve to your guests? Delicious and addictive, it's also perfect for canning.

Makes about 4 cups

7 cups fresh tomatoes, chopped

2 large onions, chopped

1 red bell pepper, chopped

1 green bell pepper, chopped

2 jalapeño peppers,
  seeded and chopped

¼ cup apple cider vinegar

2 garlic cloves, minced

¼ cup chopped fresh cilantro

1. Place the tomatoes, onions, red bell pepper, green bell pepper, jalapeños, vinegar, and garlic in a 6-quart slow cooker. Stir to combine.

2. Cover and cook on low for 7 to 8 hours, or until the vegetables are tender.

3. In batches, spoon the tomato mixture and the cilantro into a blender or food processor. Pulse until you achieve your desired thickness.

4. Refrigerate leftovers.

Per Serving (½ cup): Calories: 62; Total Fat: 0g; Saturated Fat: 0g; Trans Fat: 0g; Polyunsaturated Fat: 0g; Monounsaturated Fat: 0g; Cholesterol: 0mg; Sodium: 15mg; Carbohydrates: 13g; Fiber: 3g; Sugars: 7g; Protein: 2g

COOKING TIP: The oils from jalapeños can burn your skin, so use disposable gloves when handling and avoid touching your face.

HOMEMADE KETCHUP

Prep time: 5 minutes / Cook time: 7 to 8 hours on low

This recipe is such a simple way to make fresh ketchup. It can be customized to your taste, yet takes very little work. Just a few ingredients like tomatoes, spices, honey, and sugar placed into your slow cooker for several hours produces a big batch of ketchup that you may find yourself putting on everything!

Makes 3 to 4 cups

4 pounds tomatoes, seeded and chopped

⅔ cup apple cider vinegar

½ cup chopped onion

¼ cup brown sugar

1 teaspoon smoked paprika

1 teaspoon garlic powder

½ teaspoon celery seed

½ teaspoon freshly ground black pepper

½ teaspoon salt

⅛ teaspoon ground mustard powder

1. Combine all the ingredients in a 6-quart slow cooker. Cover and cook on low for 7 to 8 hours or until the ketchup has reduced and thickened.

2. Use an immersion blender or transfer to a food processor or blender to purée the ketchup to your desired consistency.

3. Place the ketchup in resealable jars or other airtight containers. Cool completely, then seal and refrigerate.

Per Serving (2 tablespoons): Calories: 23; Total Fat: 0g; Saturated Fat: 0g; Trans Fat: 0g; Polyunsaturated Fat: 0g; Monounsaturated Fat: 0g; Cholesterol: 0mg; Sodium: 56mg; Carbohydrates: 6g; Fiber: 1g; Sugars: 4g; Protein: 1g

SUBSTITUTION TIP: If tomatoes aren't in season, replace the fresh tomatoes with two 28-ounce cans of whole peeled tomatoes.

CREAMY QUESO DIP

Prep time: 5 minutes / Cook time: 4 hours on low

This heart-healthy Velveeta-free recipe for queso in the slow cooker is simple to prep and cook and about as nutritious as it gets when it comes to a decadent cheesy dip. You'll love the subtle sweetness and vibrant color that the butternut squash adds while keeping unhealthy fats in check. The result is a gooey and cheesy dip that is perfect for dipping vegetables or tortilla chips, or as a delicious sauce for chicken breast.

Serves 12

1 (12-ounce) bag frozen puréed butternut squash, thawed

8 ounces low-fat pepper Jack cheese or Monterey Jack, cut into cubes

8 ounces reduced-fat cream cheese

1 (4.5-ounce) can chopped green chiles

2 scallions, thinly sliced

½ cup 1% milk

½ teaspoon garlic powder

Fresh cilantro, for garnish (optional)

1. Combine the squash purée, cheese, cream cheese, chiles, scallions, milk, and garlic powder in a 6-quart slow cooker. Cover and cook on low for 4 hours or until everything is melted. Stir to combine.

2. Serve warm. Garnish with chopped fresh cilantro, if desired.

Per Serving (¼ cup): Calories: 109; Total Fat: 6g; Saturated Fat: 2g; Trans Fat: 0g; Polyunsaturated Fat: 0g; Monounsaturated Fat: 0g; Cholesterol: 23mg; Sodium: 211mg; Carbohydrates: 6g; Fiber: 0g; Sugars: 1g; Protein: 6g

SUBSTITUTION TIP: You can use a combination of pepper Jack and Monterey Jack cheeses, if you prefer. And you can replace the frozen butternut squash purée with the same amount of fresh cubed butternut squash. Place the squash cubes in a microwave-safe bowl with ½ cup of water and cook on high for 5 minutes, or until softened. Drain and mash the squash with a fork until the large pieces are broken up. Add to the slow cooker with the other ingredients as directed.

APPLE BUTTER

Prep time: 15 minutes / Cook time: 8 hours on low

This easy recipe for homemade apple butter uses simple ingredients with the best fall flavors. Aim to use sweeter apples so you can keep the amount of added sugars in check, but feel free to adjust to your liking. You can leave it slightly chunky or use an immersion blender to purée it. Use as a spread or syrup in your favorite recipes.

Makes about 2½ cups

3 pounds crisp, sweet apples, such as Fuji, Gala, Honeycrisp, or Pink Lady (about 7 medium apples), peeled, cored, and sliced

3 tablespoons pure maple syrup

2 teaspoons ground cinnamon

1 teaspoon pure vanilla extract

¼ teaspoon ground nutmeg

¼ teaspoon ground allspice

¼ teaspoon ground cloves

1. Place the apples in the bottom of a 6-quart slow cooker, then top them with the maple syrup, cinnamon, vanilla, nutmeg, allspice, and cloves. Mix well. Cover and cook on low for 8 hours. The finished apple butter should be thick and dark brown.

2. If desired, use an immersion blender or transfer to a stand blender to purée until smooth.

3. Cover and refrigerate for up to 2 weeks or freeze in small airtight containers.

Per Serving (2 tablespoons): Calories: 53; Total Fat: 0g; Saturated Fat: 0g; Trans Fat: 0g; Polyunsaturated Fat: 0g; Monounsaturated Fat: 0g; Cholesterol: 0mg; Sodium: 1mg; Carbohydrates: 14g; Fiber: 2g; Sugars: 11g; Protein: 0g

NUTRITIONAL HIGHLIGHT: Apples are heart-healthy! They lower cholesterol thanks to their high amounts of pectin, a soluble fiber that lowers cholesterol levels naturally.

CRANBERRY SAUCE

Prep time: 5 minutes / Cook time: 3 to 4 hours on high or 7 to 8 hours on low

Slow cooker cranberry sauce couldn't be easier and tastes so much better than the store-bought canned variety. You just toss the ingredients in, give it a stir, and let it make the whole house smell amazing. Feel free to jazz it up with whatever you like—cinnamon sticks, black peppercorns, vanilla extract—the possibilities are endless.

Makes about 1½ cups

12 ounces fresh cranberries

½ cup 100% orange juice

½ cup water

⅓ cup sugar (use your desired kind of sugar or sweetener, add more or less to taste)

1. Combine the ingredients in a 6-quart slow cooker. Cover and cook on high for 3 to 4 hours or on low for 7 to 8 hours, or until the cranberries have popped open and the sauce is bubbly.

2. Taste and stir in any extra sweetener or any other add-ins of your choice, such as orange zest, a pinch of ground ginger, a pinch of cinnamon or cloves, or a splash of vanilla extract. Serve warm.

Per Serving (½ cup): Calories: 155; Total Fat: 0g; Saturated Fat: 0g; Trans Fat: 0g; Polyunsaturated Fat: 0g; Monounsaturated Fat: 0g; Cholesterol: 0mg; Sodium: 3mg; Carbohydrates: 40g; Fiber: 5g; Sugars: 30g; Protein: 1g

COOKING TIP: The sauce will look a little thin when it's done and you may be tempted to cook it longer but don't. When the cranberry sauce starts cooling, the natural pectin in the cranberries helps thicken the sauce to the perfect consistency.

SAVORY VEGETABLE BROTH

Prep time: 10 minutes / Cook time: 4 hours on high or 8 hours on low

Making your own broths helps cut out sodium and fat. Even though this recipe includes a bit of salt to keep the broth full of flavor, it eliminates more than half the amount of sodium found in most store-bought reduced-sodium broths.

Makes 12 cups

12 cups water

1 (14-ounce) can no-salt-added diced tomatoes

3 carrots, sliced

4 celery stalks, sliced

4 small potatoes, cut into chunks

1 onion, cut into chunks

1 cup mushrooms, roughly chopped

4 to 6 garlic cloves, peeled and smashed

1 bunch flat leaf parsley

1 tablespoon extra-virgin olive oil

1 tablespoon Mrs. Dash

2 teaspoons Italian seasoning

¾ teaspoon salt

½ teaspoon freshly ground black pepper

2 bay leaves

1. Combine all the ingredients in a 6-quart slow cooker. Cover with the lid and cook on high for 4 hours or low for 8 hours.

2. Pour the broth through a fine-mesh strainer, discarding the solids. Refrigerate in an airtight container for up to 5 days or freeze in 1- to 2-cup portions in airtight containers.

Per Serving (1 cup): Calories: 33; Total Fat: 1g; Saturated Fat: 0g; Trans Fat: 0g; Polyunsaturated Fat: 0g; Monounsaturated Fat: 0g; Cholesterol: 0mg; Sodium: 154mg; Carbohydrates: 6g; Fiber: 3g; Sugars: 3g; Protein: 0g

COOKING TIP: This recipe can double as a vegetable soup. Leave all the veggies in the broth, but remove the bay leaves and parsley before serving.

CHICKEN STOCK

Prep time: 5 minutes / Cook time: 7 to 8 hours on low

You will be amazed at how good homemade stock tastes if you are used to the taste of canned or boxed stocks. Use this simple, fresh, and delicious stock in your favorite soup or stew recipes or freeze in 2-cup portions for later use. Since you control the ingredients, you know it contains no unnecessary additives or excessive amounts of salt.

Makes 6 to 6½ cups

2½ pounds bone-in
   chicken pieces

Water to cover, about 8 cups

2 celery stalks, chopped

2 carrots, chopped

1 onion, quartered

1 bay leaf

1 tablespoon dried basil

1 teaspoon black peppercorns

⅛ teaspoon salt

1. Combine all of the ingredients in a 6-quart slow cooker. Cover and cook on low for 7 to 8 hours.

2. Strain before using, discarding the vegetables. The chicken may be removed from the bones and used in soup.

3. The stock will thicken as it cools. Use immediately, or freeze the stock in 1- to 2-cup portions in airtight containers for up to 3 months.

Per Serving (1 cup): Calories: 35; Total Fat: 0g; Saturated Fat: 0g; Trans Fat: 0g; Polyunsaturated Fat: 0g; Monounsaturated Fat: 0g; Cholesterol: 0mg; Sodium: 111mg; Carbohydrates: 4g; Fiber: 0g; Sugars: 2g; Protein: 3g

COOKING TIP: Stock is technically different from broth because stock always involves bones, while broth does not.

TURKEY STOCK

Prep time: 10 minutes / Cook time: 8 to 12 hours on low

Don't let the hard work of cooking a whole turkey go to waste—with just a few minutes of prep you can be on your way to making your own turkey stock for use in your favorite recipes. You can change this recipe based on what vegetables and herbs you have on hand. The use of the slow cooker makes the process virtually effortless.

Makes 8 cups

Bones, skin, drippings from
   a roast turkey carcass
2 carrots, cut into chunks
2 celery ribs, cut into chunks
1 onion or leek, chopped
2 bay leaves
2 or 3 fresh sage or thyme sprigs
½ teaspoon salt
Water to cover, about 10 cups

1. Place the turkey bones, skin, and drippings; carrots; celery; onion; bay leaves; sage; and salt in a 6-quart slow cooker. Add the water. Cover and cook on low for 8 to 12 hours.

2. Let the stock cool, then strain it through a fine-mesh strainer, pressing on the solids to release all liquid. Discard the solids.

3. Chill the stock in the refrigerator. As the fat rises to the top and solidifies, you can remove and discard this.

4. Use the stock in your recipes or freeze in 1- or 2-cup portions in airtight containers for up to 3 months.

Per Serving (1 cup): Calories: 37; Total Fat: 2g; Saturated Fat: 1g; Trans Fat: 0g; Polyunsaturated Fat: 0g; Monounsaturated Fat: 1g; Cholesterol: 7mg; Sodium: 196mg; Carbohydrates: 3g; Fiber: 0g; Sugars: 1g; Protein: 2g

VARIATION TIP: You can vary this recipe by using fish bones to make a fish stock. Simply use about 2 pounds of fish bones and shrimp shells in place of the turkey carcass and add a 14-ounce can of diced tomatoes and splash of lemon juice for a deep rich flavor.

BEEF STOCK

Prep time: 15 minutes / Cook time: 8 hours on low

Slow cooking beef bones causes the bones and ligaments to release compounds like collagen and other nutrients to create a broth that has been said to have a number of beneficial effects, including reduced joint pain and inflammation. You don't have to roast the bones before adding to the pot, but do it if you have the time; roasting results in a richer flavor.

Makes 8 cups

3 pounds beef bones,
   or more to taste
3 carrots, chopped
2 celery stalks, chopped
1 onion, chopped
4 garlic cloves, smashed
1 teaspoon black peppercorns
2 bay leaves
Water to cover, about 10 cups
2 tablespoons apple
   cider vinegar

1. Optional step: Preheat oven to 375°F. Line a baking sheet with aluminum foil and spread the beef bones on the baking sheet. Roast the bones until browned, 25 to 30 minutes.

2. Place the carrots, celery, onion, garlic, peppercorns, and bay leaves in a slow cooker. Place the bones over the vegetables. Pour in enough water to cover the bones. Add the vinegar. Cover and cook on low for 8 hours.

3. Pour the stock through a fine-mesh strainer into a bowl and discard any strained solids.

4. Freeze in 1- or 2-cup portions in airtight containers for up to 3 months.

Per Serving (1 cup): Calories: 39; Total Fat: 3g; Saturated Fat: 2g; Trans Fat: 0g; Polyunsaturated Fat: 0g; Monounsaturated Fat: 1g; Cholesterol: 7mg; Sodium: 196mg; Carbohydrates: 1g; Fiber: 0g; Sugars: 1g; Protein: 2g

NUTRITIONAL HIGHLIGHT: You want your broth to gel as it cools, as this gel contains the collagen with its nutritional benefits. Try to use bones from grass-fed and pastured animals, because the type of fat in those bones will provide the most health benefits.

SLOW-COOKED BEANS

Prep time: Presoak overnight / Cook time: 7 to 8 hours on low

If you've ever cooked dried beans from scratch, you know they cook fairly easily on the stove, but you're tied to watching the pot for at least 2 hours. Using the slow cooker means you don't have to stand around in the kitchen for hours, which will free up your valuable time. Cooking beans from scratch is also less expensive than buying canned, and making a big batch means you can freeze the extra until you are ready to use them.

Makes 6 cups

1 pound dried beans
Water

1. Rinse the beans in a colander and allow to drain.

2. Pour the beans into a 6-quart slow cooker and add enough water to cover beans by 2 inches, about 6 to 8 cups. Let the beans soak for at least 6 hours or overnight. Do not turn the slow cooker on.

3. Rinse and drain the beans again. Return them to the slow cooker and cover with fresh water as in step 2. Cover and cook on low for 7 to 8 hours, or until softened.

4. Drain the beans and let them cool. Freeze them in resealable bags. About 1⅔ cups of cooked beans is the equivalent of a 14.5-ounce can of beans.

Per Serving (1 cup): Calories: 259; Total Fat: 0g; Saturated Fat: 0g; Trans Fat: 0g; Polyunsaturated Fat: 0g; Monounsaturated Fat: 0g; Cholesterol: 0mg; Sodium: 11mg; Carbohydrates: 48g; Fiber: 11g; Sugars: 2g; Protein: 15g

COOKING TIP: Every bean is different, so the cooking time will vary depending on the bean. As a general rule, set the timer for the lower end of the range and check for doneness.

MUSHROOM GRAVY

Prep time: 5 minutes / Cook time: 5 to 8 hours on low

This versatile vegetarian gravy is quick to prep and can be used on any of your favorite dishes. The best kind of gravy is homemade!

Makes about 2 cups

1 cup button mushrooms, sliced

¾ cup low-fat buttermilk

⅓ cup water

1 medium onion, finely diced

2 garlic cloves, minced

2 tablespoons extra-virgin olive oil

2 tablespoons all-purpose flour

1 tablespoon fresh rosemary, minced

Freshly ground black pepper

1. Combine all of the ingredients in a 6-quart slow cooker. Cover and cook on low 5 to 8 hours.

2. Serve warm. Refrigerate leftovers in an airtight container for 3 or 4 days, or freeze for up to 4 months.

Per Serving (¼ cup): Calories: 54; Total Fat: 4g; Saturated Fat: 1g; Trans Fat: 0g; Polyunsaturated Fat: 1g; Monounsaturated Fat: 2g; Cholesterol: 0mg; Sodium: 25mg; Carbohydrates: 4g; Fiber: 1g; Sugars: 2g; Protein: 2g

SUBSTITUTION TIP: You can make delicious gluten-free mushroom gravy by replacing the flour with cornstarch.

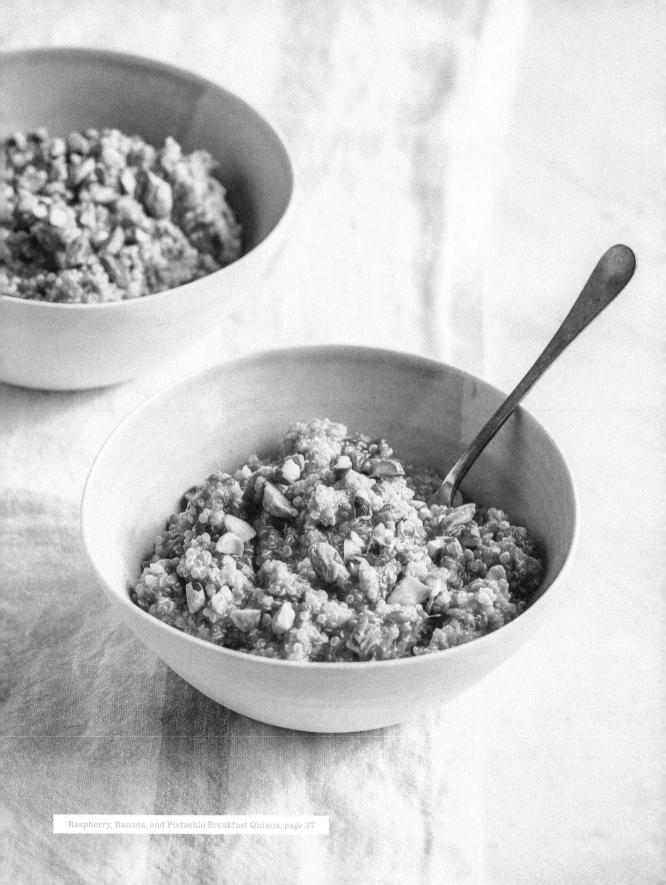

Raspberry, Banana, and Pistachio Breakfast Quinoa, page 37

3

Breakfasts

VEGETABLE FRITTATA

Prep time: 10 minutes / Cook time: 6 to 8 hours on low

This breakfast frittata is all about traditional breakfast flavors: potatoes, eggs, and cheese. The preparation involves some chopping and whisking the eggs, but then you just add everything to your slow cooker and you are all set.

Serves 8

Nonstick cooking spray

2 medium sweet potatoes, thinly sliced

½ cup canned light coconut milk

¼ cup water

2 large bell peppers, chopped

1 medium onion, chopped

1 cup chopped kale

12 large eggs, whisked

4 ounces shredded low-fat Swiss cheese

Freshly ground black pepper

1. Spray the inside of a 6-quart slow cooker with the cooking spray. Place the sweet potato slices on the bottom of the slow cooker and pour the coconut milk over them.

2. Next layer the chopped bell peppers, onion, and kale. Pour the eggs on top. Add the cheese and season with black pepper. Cover and cook on low for 6 to 8 hours, or until the eggs are set.

3. Serve hot.

Per Serving (approximately 1 cup): Calories: 215; Total Fat: 11g; Saturated Fat: 5g; Trans Fat: 0g; Polyunsaturated Fat: 2g; Monounsaturated Fat: 3g; Cholesterol: 289mg; Sodium: 188mg; Carbohydrates: 13g; Fiber: 3g; Sugars: 8g; Protein: 15g

> VARIATION TIP: You can use whatever vegetables you have on hand and your favorite herbs and spices. You could also add cooked beans for a fiber and protein boost.

CARAMELIZED APPLE CINNAMON OATS

Prep time: 10 minutes / Cook time: 7 to 8 hours on low

This breakfast of apple cinnamon oatmeal tastes like apple pie with its sweet caramel goodness. Made with natural sweeteners that are adaptable to your personal tastes, all it takes is a few minutes of prep time for you to wake up to a heart-healthy, filling, and delicious breakfast.

Serves 6

Nonstick cooking spray

2 pounds apples (about 5 large or 9 small apples), chopped into 1-inch pieces (peeling is optional)

½ cup brown sugar (more or less to taste)

1 tablespoon ground cinnamon

½ teaspoon ground nutmeg

2 tablespoons freshly squeezed lemon juice

Pinch salt

2 cups rolled oats

2 large eggs

2 cups low-fat or fat-free milk, or plant-based milk

1½ cups water

1. Generously grease the bowl of a 6-quart slow cooker with the cooking spray.

2. In a large bowl, add the apples, brown sugar, cinnamon, nutmeg, lemon juice, and salt and toss to combine. Add the oats and stir again. Pour the mixture into the slow cooker.

3. Using the same bowl, whisk the eggs into the milk until the mixture is very smooth. Add the water and whisk again. Pour this mixture over the apple-oat mixture. Cover and cook on low for 7 to 8 hours.

4. Serve warm.

Per Serving (approximately 1½ cups): Calories: 202; Total Fat: 4g; Saturated Fat: 1g; Trans Fat: 0g; Polyunsaturated Fat: 1g; Monounsaturated Fat: 1g; Cholesterol: 67mg; Sodium: 95mg; Carbohydrates: 36g; Fiber: 4g; Sugars: 24g; Protein: 8g

COOKING TIP: To caramelize the apples even more, skip the tossing in step 2 and instead layer the apples, brown sugar, salt, cinnamon, nutmeg, lemon juice, and oats in the greased pot in that order and do not stir. Whisk the milk, eggs, and water as in step 3 and pour over the layered apples. Cook as directed.

VARIATION TIP: You can make this recipe gluten-free by using gluten-free rolled oats.

BLUEBERRY-WALNUT STEEL-CUT OATMEAL

Prep time: 5 minutes / Cook time: 7 to 8 hours on low

This oatmeal recipe is full of cholesterol-lowering fiber and energy-sustaining complex carbohydrates. Steel-cut oats are minimally processed, so they are perfect for the slow cooker. There's no better way to start your day than with oats, blueberries, and a ripe banana for added sweetness.

Serves 8

Nonstick cooking spray

2 cups steel-cut oats

6 cups water

2 cups low-fat or fat-free milk, or plant-based milk

2 cups fresh or frozen blueberries

1 ripe banana, mashed

1 teaspoon vanilla extract

2 teaspoons ground cinnamon

2 tablespoons brown sugar

Pinch salt

½ cup chopped walnuts, for garnish

1. Spray the bowl of the slow cooker with the cooking spray.

2. Place the oats, water, milk, blueberries, banana, vanilla, cinnamon, brown sugar, and salt in the slow cooker. Stir well. Cover and cook on low for 7 to 8 hours.

3. Serve warm garnished with the chopped walnuts.

Per Serving (approximately 1½ cups): Calories: 202; Total Fat: 4g; Saturated Fat: 1g; Trans Fat: 0g; Polyunsaturated Fat: 1g; Monounsaturated Fat: 1g; Cholesterol: 67mg; Sodium: 95mg; Carbohydrates: 36g; Fiber: 4g; Sugars: 24g; Protein: 8g

COOKING TIP: When you make oatmeal in your slow cooker the first time, I suggest you monitor the time it takes to cook it to your desired consistency. Slow cookers vary greatly in their heat intensity. To prevent burnt edges, always spray the inside with cooking spray or consider using a slow cooker liner.

VARIATION TIP: You can make this recipe gluten-free by using gluten-free steel-cut oats.

CREAMY BANANA FRENCH TOAST

Prep time: 10 minutes / Cook time: 4 to 5 hours on low

You don't need to limit yourself to making slow cooker oats or an eggs-and-potato casserole for breakfast. This easy, creamy, and nutritious banana French toast recipe will shake up your morning routine with fiber-rich bread and potassium-rich bananas. Simply plate the French toast and drizzle with your favorite syrup or sauce.

Serves 6

Nonstick cooking spray

12 (1-inch) slices whole-wheat baguette

4 large eggs

¾ cup low-fat or fat-free milk, or unsweetened almond milk

1 tablespoon brown sugar

1 tablespoon vanilla extract

1 teaspoon ground cinnamon

2 ripe bananas, sliced

Juice of ½ lemon

2 tablespoons dairy-free or trans fat–free soft margarine or coconut oil, melted

½ cup chopped walnuts or nut of choice

1. Spray the bowl of a 6-quart slow cooker with the cooking spray. Arrange the baguette slices on the bottom of the slow cooker.

2. Whisk together the eggs, milk, sugar, vanilla, and cinnamon. Pour this over the baguette slices, making sure to cover each slice completely with the egg mixture.

3. In a medium mixing bowl, cover the banana slices with the lemon juice, tossing to coat. Place the banana slices atop the baguettes in the slow cooker. Drizzle with the melted margarine and sprinkle with the walnuts. Cover and cook on low for 4 to 5 hours, or until cooked through.

4. Serve warm.

Per Serving (2 slices bread plus ⅓ cup toppings): Calories: 273; Total Fat: 11g; Saturated Fat: 3g; Trans Fat: 0g; Polyunsaturated Fat: 6g; Monounsaturated Fat: 4g; Cholesterol: 125mg; Sodium: 278mg; Carbohydrates: 33g; Fiber: 5g; Sugars: 10g; Protein: 12g

NUTRITIONAL HIGHLIGHT: Bananas are one of the most nutritious foods you can include in your diet for heart health. Bananas are an excellent source of potassium, a mineral that regulates fluid levels in the body. Potassium can lower blood pressure and reduce the effects of sodium on blood pressure.

BREAKFAST BARLEY

Prep time: 5 minutes / Cook time: 7 to 8 hours on low

Move over oats and whole-grain bread: Make room for barley. This soft, spherical grain is rich in a slow-digesting carbohydrate that keeps your blood sugar levels steadier than other grains. It is also an excellent source of the cholesterol-lowering fiber beta-glucan. This simple-to-prep recipe is easy to customize to your tastes and will leave you feeling full for hours.

Serves 6

7 cups water

2 cups hulled barley, rinsed well

1. Put the water and the barley in a 6-quart slow cooker. Stir well. Cover and cook on low for 7 to 8 hours.

2. Serve warm with toppings such as fresh fruit, cinnamon, a dash vanilla extract, low-fat or plant-based milk, or chopped nuts. Refrigerate any leftovers in an airtight container for up to 5 days.

Per Serving (1¼ cups): Calories: 217; Total Fat: 1g; Saturated Fat: 0g; Trans Fat: 0g; Polyunsaturated Fat: 0g; Monounsaturated Fat: 0g; Cholesterol: 7mg; Sodium: 7mg; Carbohydrates: 45g; Fiber: 11g; Sugars: 0g; Protein: 8g

VARIATION TIP: This recipe is kept simple on purpose so that one batch of barley can be eaten and shared in many different ways throughout the week without boredom. Flavor combinations to try include strawberries and milk, banana nut, cherry almond, and mango coconut.

RASPBERRY, BANANA, AND PISTACHIO BREAKFAST QUINOA

Prep time: 10 minutes / Cook time: 7 to 8 hours on low

This recipe is the perfect way to start your busy mornings. Quinoa is a complete plant protein, meaning it has all of the amino acids your body needs, plus ample vitamins and minerals. Raspberries, bananas, and pistachios all boost its nutrition and heart health benefits by adding fiber, potassium, and healthy fats. This breakfast will keep you feeling full and energized until lunchtime.

Serves 8

2½ cups low-fat or fat-free milk, or plant-based milk

2 cups water

2 cups quinoa, rinsed and drained

2 cups frozen raspberries

1 medium ripe banana, mashed

1 tablespoon honey

1 teaspoon ground cinnamon

1 cup shelled pistachios, chopped, for garnish

1. Combine the milk, water, quinoa, raspberries, banana, honey, and cinnamon in a 6-quart slow cooker. Cover and cook on low for 7 to 8 hours.

2. Serve hot, garnished with the chopped pistachios.

Per Serving (1¼ cups): Calories: 297; Total Fat: 8g; Saturated Fat: 1g; Trans Fat: 0g; Polyunsaturated Fat: 4g; Monounsaturated Fat: 5g; Cholesterol: 4mg; Sodium: 39mg; Carbohydrates: 54g; Fiber: 7g; Sugars: 22g; Protein: 10g

COOKING TIP: Quinoa has a natural coating called saponin, which can make it taste bitter. That is why it is often recommended that this seed be rinsed before using. Boxed quinoa is usually prerinsed, but it can't hurt to rinse it again before using.

ALMOND RICE BREAKFAST PUDDING

Prep time: 10 minutes / Cook time: 6 to 8 hours on low

Brown rice makes a warm, filling, and nourishing breakfast. Many other cultures incorporate this healthy grain into breakfast. By omitting eggs, cream, and large amounts of sugar, this lightly sweetened breakfast pudding is an energizing alternative to your standard breakfast.

Serves 8

Nonstick cooking spray

6 cups low-fat or fat-free milk, or plant-based milk

2 cups long-grain brown rice

1 cup raisins

1 ripe banana, mashed

1 tablespoon honey, maple syrup, or sweetener of choice

2 teaspoons vanilla extract

1 teaspoon ground cinnamon

½ cup chopped almonds

1. Spray the inside of a 6-quart slow cooker with the cooking spray. Combine the milk, rice, raisins, banana, honey, vanilla, and cinnamon. Cover and cook on low for 6 to 8 hours.

2. Serve hot. Top the rice with the chopped almonds and additional milk and sweetener, if desired.

Per Serving (1 cup): Calories: 393; Total Fat: 8g; Saturated Fat: 2g; Trans Fat: 0g; Polyunsaturated Fat: 1g; Monounsaturated Fat: 2g; Cholesterol: 11mg; Sodium: 115mg; Carbohydrates: 68g; Fiber: 4g; Sugars: 16g; Protein: 14g

VARIATION TIP: For additional heart-healthy omega-3 fatty acids and fiber, consider adding 2 tablespoons of chia seeds or ground flaxseed to the slow cooker with the other ingredients.

POTATO, PEPPER, AND EGG BREAKFAST CASSEROLE

Prep time: 10 minutes / Cook time: 7 to 8 hours on low

Any time you can start your day with vegetables is a great day. This vegetarian breakfast casserole is an all-in-one dish that is filling and heart-healthy. Have guests in from out of town? Spend more time visiting and less time cooking! Thaw the hash browns in the refrigerator during the day and put them in the slow cooker that night. You will wake up to a delicious meal that everyone will enjoy.

Serves 8

12 large eggs

1 cup low-fat milk

¼ teaspoon dried mustard

½ teaspoon garlic powder

½ teaspoon salt

½ teaspoon freshly ground black pepper

Nonstick cooking spray

1 (30-ounce) bag frozen hash browns, thawed in the refrigerator

1 (14-ounce) bag frozen peppers and onions, thawed in the refrigerator

6 ounces (1½ cups) 2% shredded Cheddar cheese

1. In a large bowl, whisk together the eggs, milk, dried mustard, garlic powder, salt, and pepper.

2. Spray the bowl a 6-quart slow cooker with the cooking spray. Layer one-third of the hash browns in the slow cooker followed by one-third of the peppers and onions, then one-third of the cheese. Repeat the layers two more times.

3. Slowly pour the egg mixture over the top. Cover and cook on low for 7 to 8 hours.

4. Cut into 8 wedges and serve hot.

Per Serving (1 wedge): Calories: 340; Total Fat: 18g; Saturated Fat: 6g; Trans Fat: 0g; Polyunsaturated Fat: 2g; Monounsaturated Fat: 3g; Cholesterol: 296mg; Sodium: 421mg; Carbohydrates: 27g; Fiber: 3g; Sugars: 3g; Protein: 20g

COOKING TIP: Allowing the hash browns and vegetables to thaw before they are added to the slow cooker keeps the ingredients out of the temperature "danger zone" of 40°F to 140°F so they remain safe to eat. Drain off any excess water before proceeding with the recipe.

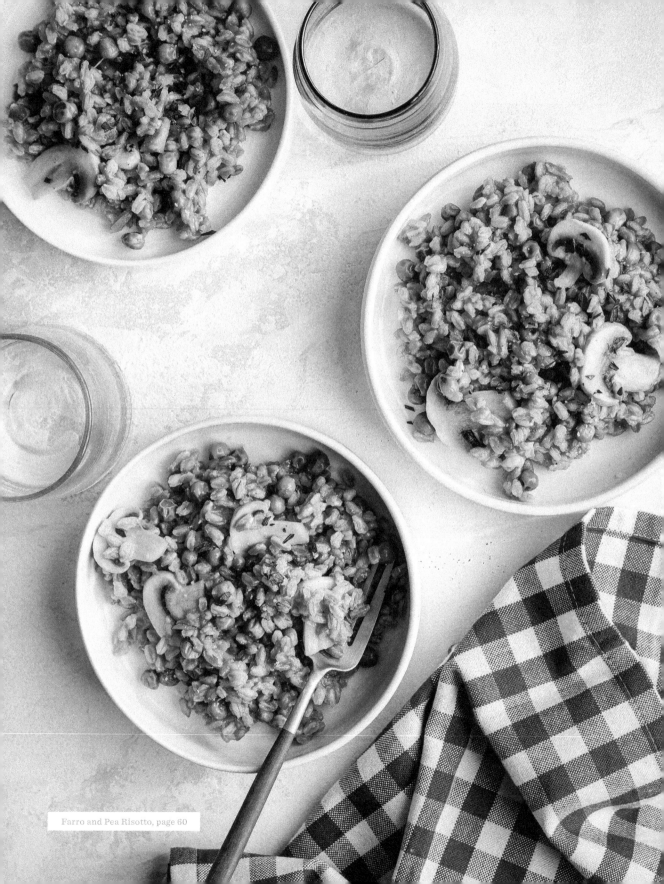

Farro and Pea Risotto, page 60

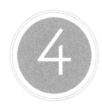

Beans and Grains

WHEAT BERRY–EDAMAME PILAF

Prep time: 5 minutes / Cook time: 6 to 8 hours on low

This hearty vegetarian dish is packed with whole grains and complete protein. Edamame are green soybeans, a high-quality vegetarian source of protein rich in beneficial plant phytonutrients and filling fiber. They also make a fantastic snack. Just thaw, throw some in a container, and you have a nutritious snack on the go.

Serves 12

1 cup wheat berries

1 cup wild rice

4 cups Savory Vegetable Broth (page 24) or low-sodium vegetable broth

2 cups frozen shelled edamame

1 medium red bell pepper, chopped

1 red onion, finely chopped

4 garlic cloves, minced

1 tablespoon extra-virgin olive oil

1 teaspoon dried thyme

Freshly ground black pepper

1. Rinse and drain the wheat berries and wild rice.

2. In a 6-quart slow cooker, combine the broth, edamame, wheat berries, wild rice, bell pepper, onion, garlic, olive oil, and thyme. Season with the pepper. Cover and cook on low for 6 to 8 hours on low until the liquid is absorbed.

3. Serve hot, with a green salad.

Per Serving (⅔ cup): Calories: 168; Total Fat: 3g; Saturated Fat: 1g; Trans Fat: 0g; Polyunsaturated Fat: 1g; Monounsaturated Fat: 1g; Cholesterol: 0mg; Sodium: 50mg; Carbohydrates: 28g; Fiber: 5g; Sugars: 1g; Protein: 9g

NUTRITIONAL HIGHLIGHT: Wheat berries are whole-wheat kernels that look like thick, short rice grains similar to brown rice. Since the kernel is left intact, this grain is rich in nutrients and packed with fiber, protein, and iron.

SPICY CREOLE BLACK-EYED PEAS

Prep time: 5 minutes / Cook time: 7 to 8 hours on low

This vegan recipe for spicy Creole black-eyed peas can be an entry in your "easy and awesome" recipe category. With no added fats, this fiber- and protein-rich dish gets its flavor and spice from the addition of vegetables, Creole seasonings, and diced jalapeños. Serve this creamy and nutritious dish over whole-grain rice.

Serves 8

6 cups Savory Vegetable Broth (page 24) or low-sodium vegetable broth

1 pound dried black-eyed peas

6 celery stalks, chopped

2 medium tomatoes, diced

1 (4-ounce) can diced jalapeño peppers

1 onion, diced

6 garlic cloves, minced

1 or 2 canned chipotle peppers in adobo sauce, chopped

1 tablespoon freshly squeezed lemon juice

1 tablespoon Creole seasoning, or more to taste

1. Put all of the ingredients in a 6-quart slow cooker and stir to combine. Cover and cook on low for 7 to 8 hours.

2. Serve warm over brown rice.

Per Serving (1 cup): Calories: 177; Total Fat: 0g; Saturated Fat: 0g; Trans Fat: 0g; Polyunsaturated Fat: 0g; Monounsaturated Fat: 0g; Cholesterol: 0mg; Sodium: 286mg; Carbohydrates: 43g; Fiber: 18g; Sugars: 5g; Protein: 15g

> NUTRITIONAL HIGHLIGHT: Black-eyed peas are actually a legume and get their name from their appearance. This nutrient-rich bean is one of the few beans that doesn't require presoaking and it's high in fiber, the blood pressure–regulating mineral potassium, B vitamins, protein, and iron.

BEST-EVER BAKED BEANS

Prep time: 10 minutes, plus overnight to soak / Cook time: 7 to 8 hours on low

Most traditional baked beans are made with bacon, but you won't miss it in this vegan version of Boston baked beans, which uses smoky paprika to give you the taste you crave. Beans are an ideal side dish for summer barbecues; you can skip the processed canned variety as these could not be any easier to make from scratch.

Serves 8

1 pound dry navy beans, soaked overnight (see Cooking Tip)

6 cups Savory Vegetable Broth (page 24) or water

1 large sweet onion, diced

1 medium yellow bell pepper, diced

½ cup Homemade Ketchup (page 20)

¼ cup maple syrup

2 tablespoons molasses

1 tablespoon extra-virgin olive oil

1 teaspoon dried mustard

¼ teaspoon garlic powder

2 teaspoons smoked paprika

1 tablespoon apple cider vinegar

Freshly ground black pepper

1. Drain and rinse the soaked beans and put them in a 6-quart slow cooker. Stir in the broth, onion, bell pepper, ketchup, maple syrup, molasses, olive oil, dried mustard, garlic powder, and paprika. Cover and cook on low for 7 to 8 hours.

2. Stir in the vinegar and season with the pepper just before serving.

Per Serving (1 cup): Calories: 295; Total Fat: 2g; Saturated Fat: 0g; Trans Fat: 0g; Polyunsaturated Fat: 0g; Monounsaturated Fat: 1g; Cholesterol: 0mg; Sodium: 113mg; Carbohydrates: 55g; Fiber: 16g; Sugars: 18g; Protein: 13g

COOKING TIP: To ensure even cooking, soak the dried beans before slow cooking. Place the beans in a large pot or the slow cooker bowl, cover with cold water, and soak at room temperature overnight, or for at least 8 hours. Drain and rinse before using.

LIMA BEAN CASSEROLE

Prep time: 5 minutes, plus overnight to soak / Cook time: 7 to 8 hours on low

Sometimes called "butter beans" because of their starchy yet buttery texture, lima beans have a delicate flavor that complements a wide variety of dishes. This meat-free version pairs this nutritious bean with sweet potato, tomatoes, and carrots. It's delicious served with some homemade cornbread.

Serves 8

1 pound dried lima beans, soaked overnight

1 (28-ounce) can no-salt-added tomatoes, diced

1 cup finely chopped sweet potato

1 medium carrot, finely chopped

1 onion, finely chopped

4 garlic cloves, minced

1 tablespoon dried mustard

½ teaspoon freshly ground black pepper

2 cups water

1. Rinse the soaked beans in cold water and drain.

2. Put the beans in a 6-quart slow cooker along with the tomatoes, sweet potato, carrot, onion, garlic, dried mustard, pepper, and water. Be certain that the water fully covers the ingredients; add more if needed. Stir to combine. Cover and cook on low for 7 to 8 hours.

3. Serve warm.

Per Serving (1¼ cups): Calories: 153; Total Fat: 0g; Saturated Fat: 0g; Trans Fat: 0g; Polyunsaturated Fat: 0g; Monounsaturated Fat: 0g; Cholesterol: 0mg; Sodium: 40mg; Carbohydrates: 44g; Fiber: 24g; Sugars: 9g; Protein: 14g

SUBSTITUTION TIP: For a more traditional nonvegan lima bean recipe, replace the sweet potato with 1 cup of diced ham, turkey ham, or chicken-and-apple sausage.

ALLERGY-FREE • VEGAN

SWEET-AND-SOUR BEANS

Prep time: 5 minutes, plus overnight to soak / Cook time: 7 to 8 hours on low

Combining sweet and sour flavors may make you think of pork and other meat dishes, but the flavors work wonderfully for beans, as well. Dried white beans are used in this recipe, but you can use the beans of your choice. The beans freeze very well so you can make a big batch and keep some on hand as a great side dish for future meals.

Serves 8

1 pound white beans, soaked overnight

4 cups Savory Vegetable Broth (page 24) or low-sodium vegetable broth

1 (6-ounce) can no-salt-added tomato paste

1 cup water

3 carrots, diced

1 sweet onion, diced

2 red, orange, yellow, or green bell peppers, diced

¼ cup Homemade Ketchup (page 20)

¼ cup dry cooking sherry

¼ cup low-sodium tamari

¼ cup cider vinegar

2 tablespoons sugar

1 tablespoon dried marjoram

1 tablespoon dried thyme

2 teaspoons freshly ground black pepper

1 tablespoon cornstarch or arrowroot

1. Drain and rinse the beans. Put them in a 6-quart slow cooker along with the broth, tomato paste, water, carrots, onion, bell peppers, ketchup, sherry, tamari, vinegar, sugar, marjoram, thyme, and pepper. Cover and cook on low for 7 to 8 hours.

2. With 15 minutes left before serving, stir in the cornstarch. Cook for another 15 minutes until the broth thickens.

3. Serve warm.

Per Serving (1¼ cups): Calories: 263; Total Fat: 0g; Saturated Fat: 0g; Trans Fat: 0g; Polyunsaturated Fat: 0g; Monounsaturated Fat: 0g; Cholesterol: 0mg; Sodium: 383mg; Carbohydrates: 49g; Fiber: 23g; Sugars: 11g; Protein: 16g

COOKING TIP: If you think you will be freezing part of this recipe, aim to use arrowroot for thickening. Unlike cornstarch, arrowroot powder creates a perfectly clear gel and does not break down when combined with acidic ingredients. Also, arrowroot stands up better to freezing, whereas mixtures thickened with cornstarch tend to break down after freezing and thawing.

ALLERGY-FREE • VEGAN

SPICY VEGAN BLACK BEAN SOUP

Prep time: 10 minutes, plus overnight to soak / Cook time: 8 to 10 hours on high

With slightly spicy undertones, this black bean soup is hearty and healthy. Top the finished soup with a bit of cilantro and a dollop of low-fat plain Greek yogurt, if you wish.

Serves 6

1 pound dried black beans

2 (14-ounce) cans no-salt-added diced tomatoes

3 cups Savory Vegetable Broth (page 24) or low-sodium vegetable broth

½ red onion, diced

1 green bell pepper, seeded and diced

1 poblano pepper, seeded and diced

2 jalapeño peppers, seeded and diced

3 tablespoons red wine vinegar

6 garlic cloves, minced

1½ tablespoons chili powder

2 teaspoons ground cumin

½ teaspoon dried oregano

½ teaspoon salt

½ teaspoon freshly ground black pepper

2 bay leaves

1. Soak the beans overnight at room temperature in a large bowl with 2 quarts of water.

2. Drain and rinse the beans and put them in a 6-quart slow cooker. Add the tomatoes, broth, onion, bell pepper, poblano, jalapeños, vinegar, garlic, chili powder, cumin, oregano, salt, pepper, and bay leaves and stir well. Cover and cook on high for 8 to 10 hours.

3. Remove the bay leaves before serving. Stir and serve hot.

Per Serving (1⅔ cups): Calories: 314; Total Fat: 0g; Saturated Fat: 0g; Trans Fat: 0g; Polyunsaturated Fat: 0g; Monounsaturated Fat: 0g; Cholesterol: 0mg; Sodium: 333mg; Carbohydrates: 60g; Fiber: 23g; Sugars: 8g; Protein: 19g

COOKING TIP: Feel free to add a pinch of cayenne for some extra heat, or scale back the spice by removing one or both of the jalapeños.

SAVORY NAVY BEAN SOUP WITH HAM

Prep time: 10 minutes, plus overnight to soak / Cook time: 8 to 10 hours on low

Bean soups definitely fit the comfort food bill and this recipe is no exception. This meal is big on fiber and flavor. A bit of slow-cooked ham elevates the taste while keeping the sodium content in check.

Serves 8

1 pound dried navy beans

2 cups Chicken Stock (page 25) or low-sodium chicken broth

1 (15-ounce) can no-salt-added diced tomatoes

8 ounces 98% fat-free, reduced-sodium ham, finely diced

3 celery ribs, diced

3 carrots, diced

1 onion, diced

3 garlic cloves, minced

1½ teaspoons onion powder

1 teaspoon dried parsley

1 teaspoon dried sage

1 teaspoon garlic powder

1 bay leaf

½ teaspoon freshly ground black pepper

½ teaspoon salt

1. Soak the beans overnight at room temperature in a large bowl with 2 quarts of water.

2. Drain and rinse the beans and put them in a 4- to 6-quart slow cooker. Cover the beans with about 1 inch of water and add the rest of the ingredients. Stir well. Cover and cook on low for 8 to 10 hours.

3. Use the back of a spoon to mash some of the beans against the sides of the slow cooker and stir them back into the soup, creating a creamier texture.

4. Serve hot.

Per Serving (1½ cups): Calories: 256; Total Fat: 0g; Saturated Fat: 0g; Trans Fat: 0g; Polyunsaturated Fat: 0g; Monounsaturated Fat: 0g; Cholesterol: 15mg; Sodium: 605mg; Carbohydrates: 44g; Fiber: 17g; Sugars: 5g; Protein: 21g

VARIATION TIP: To make this soup vegan, swap out the chicken stock for vegetable broth and eliminate the ham.

COCONUT RED BEANS AND RICE

Prep time: 5 minutes, plus overnight to soak / Cook time: 7 to 8 hours on low

When the cold of winter drags on, a filling and healthy tropical-tasting dish may be just what you need. Light coconut milk gives fiber- and protein-rich red beans a creamy, sweet consistency and tropical flair. Fresh lime juice finishes this rice and bean dish, which will elevate dinner to the extraordinary.

Serves 8

1 cup dried red beans, soaked overnight

4 cups Chicken Stock (page 25) or low-sodium chicken broth

1 (14.5-ounce) can light coconut milk

1½ cups long-grain basmati white rice

1 large onion, finely diced

2 garlic cloves, minced

1 teaspoon red pepper flakes

½ teaspoon coconut extract (optional)

1 to 2 tablespoons freshly squeezed lime juice

2 limes, cut into wedges, for serving

1. Drain and rinse the soaked beans. Add the beans to a 6-quart slow cooker along with the stock, coconut milk, rice, onion, garlic, red pepper flakes, and coconut extract (if using). Stir well. Cover and cook for 7 to 8 hours on low.

2. Just before serving, stir in the lime juice and taste to adjust seasonings.

3. Serve warm, with the lime wedges on the side.

Per Serving (1¼ cups): Calories: 262; Total Fat: 2g; Saturated Fat: 2g; Trans Fat: 0g; Polyunsaturated Fat: 0g; Monounsaturated Fat: 0g; Cholesterol: 0mg; Sodium: 99mg; Carbohydrates: 65g; Fiber: 21g; Sugars: 3g; Protein: 16g

SUBSTITUTION TIP: The chicken stock enhances the flavor of this dish because of its flavor profile; however, if you prefer a vegan dish, substitute with vegetable broth. Avoid using plain water in place of the stock, as it won't impart enough flavor.

WILD RICE MEDLEY

Prep time: 10 minutes / Cook time: 6 to 8 hours on low

A wild rice pilaf makes a wonderful bowl of nourishing comfort food during the cold winter months. Wild rice is actually a grain seed native to the Great Lakes region and parts of Canada and is higher in protein and nutrients than most other grains. Its chewy texture contrasts nicely with the meaty mushrooms in this recipe.

Serves 8

3 cups wild rice, rinsed and drained

1 tablespoon extra-virgin olive oil

6 cups Savory Vegetable Broth (page 24) or low-sodium vegetable broth

¾ cup finely chopped shallots

2 cups sliced mushrooms

2 garlic cloves, minced

1 teaspoon dried thyme

Freshly ground black pepper

½ cup chopped pecans

1 tablespoon fresh rosemary

1. Add the wild rice and oil to a 6-quart slow cooker and stir until the grains are well coated. Add the broth, shallots, mushrooms, garlic, thyme, and pepper and stir well. Cover and cook on low for 6 to 8 hours, until the rice is tender.

2. Stir in the pecans and fresh rosemary just before serving.

Per Serving (1⅓ cups): Calories: 271; Total Fat: 4g; Saturated Fat: 1g; Trans Fat: 0g; Polyunsaturated Fat: 2g; Monounsaturated Fat: 4g; Cholesterol: 0mg; Sodium: 108mg; Carbohydrates: 50g; Fiber: 5g; Sugars: 3g; Protein: 11g

NUTRITIONAL HIGHLIGHT: Wild rice is a good source of fiber, folate, and magnesium and rich in beneficial plant phytonutrients and disease-protective antioxidants.

RANCH-STYLE PINTO BEANS

Prep time: 10 minutes, plus overnight to soak / Cook time: 7 to 8 hours on low

Unlike sweeter Boston baked beans, these ranch-style pinto beans are savory with a bit of heat. Beef broth is used for a richer flavor, chili powder adds a bit of spice, and smoked paprika gives the dish a smoky flavor. The Tex-Mex flavor of these beans is a perfect pair with your favorite enchilada recipe.

Serves 8

1 pound dried pinto beans, soaked overnight

5 cups Beef Stock (page 27) or low-sodium beef broth

1 cup low-sodium tomato sauce

1 medium white onion, diced

1 jalapeño pepper, seeded, and finely diced

4 garlic cloves, minced

1 tablespoon ancho chili powder

1 teaspoon chili powder

1 teaspoon apple cider vinegar

1 teaspoon ground cumin

1 packed teaspoon brown sugar

1 teaspoon smoked paprika

½ teaspoon dried oregano

Freshly ground black pepper

1. Drain and rinse the soaked beans. Put them in a 6-quart slow cooker along with the stock, tomato sauce, onion, jalapeño, garlic, ancho chili powder, chili powder, vinegar, cumin, sugar, paprika, and oregano. Cover and cook on low for 7 to 8 hours, until the beans are tender and the liquid has thickened slightly.

2. Taste and season with the pepper. Serve warm.

Per Serving (1 cup): Calories: 222; Total Fat: 0g; Saturated Fat: 0g; Trans Fat: 0g; Polyunsaturated Fat: 0g; Monounsaturated Fat: 0g; Cholesterol: 0mg; Sodium: 290mg; Carbohydrates: 40g; Fiber: 8g; Sugars: 3g; Protein: 14g

COOKING TIP: Ancho chili powder is the go-to powder for authentic Mexican cooking. It's commonly available in the spice aisle of most supermarkets. If you can't find it, simply double the amount of regular chili powder in this recipe and add a pinch of crushed red pepper flakes.

QUINOA AND VEGETABLES

Prep time: 10 minutes / Cook time: 6 to 7 hours on low

If you are looking for a change from the usual side of rice, give this quinoa and vegetable recipe a try. Quinoa is a gluten-free seed that is a complete plant protein. It has a fluffy texture and nutty taste. This dish is easy to throw together: Simply chop a few vegetables to add to the pot and you will have a fantastic side dish that is simply delicious.

Serves 8

2 cups quinoa, rinsed and drained

4 cups Savory Vegetable Broth (page 24) or low-sodium vegetable broth

1 medium onion, chopped

1 medium red bell pepper, chopped

2 medium carrots, chopped

1 cup fresh green beans, chopped

2 garlic cloves, minced

Freshly ground black pepper

1 teaspoon chopped fresh basil, for garnish

1. Put the quinoa, broth, onion, bell pepper, carrots, green beans, garlic, and pepper in a 6-quart slow cooker. Stir to combine. Cover and cook on low for 6 to 7 hours, until the vegetables are tender and the liquid is absorbed into the quinoa.

2. Serve garnished with the fresh basil.

Per Serving (1 cup): Calories: 202; Total Fat: 3g; Saturated Fat: 0g; Trans Fat: 0g; Polyunsaturated Fat: 1g; Monounsaturated Fat: 1g; Cholesterol: 0mg; Sodium: 83mg; Carbohydrates: 38g; Fiber: 5g; Sugars: 6g; Protein: 7g

VARIATION TIP: You can make this into a complete meal by adding a can of your favorite beans (drained and rinsed) like chickpeas or black beans to the cooked quinoa and vegetables.

GARLIC VEGGIE LENTILS

Prep time: 15 minutes / Cook time: 7 to 8 hours on low

Lentils are nutritious, filling, inexpensive, and arguably the most flavorful of all legumes. There are several varieties of lentils, including green, brown, yellow, red, black (beluga), and lentilles du Puy, all of which vary slightly in taste and cooking times. For slow cooker recipes, it's best to choose du Puy or black as they will hold their shape while they cook.

Serves 8

3 cups dried lentils

5 cups Savory Vegetable Broth (page 24) or low-sodium vegetable broth

1 (28-ounce) can no-salt-added diced tomatoes

1 large onion, chopped

2 leeks, chopped

8 garlic cloves, minced

2 large carrots, chopped

2 bay leaves

1 teaspoon dried thyme

Freshly ground black pepper

1. Sort the lentils, discarding any stones or impurities. Rinse under cold water in a fine-mesh strainer.

2. Combine all of the ingredients in a 6-quart slow cooker and stir. Cover and cook on low for 7 to 8 hours until the lentils are tender and the sauce has thickened.

3. Remove and discard the bay leaf. Serve warm.

Per Serving (1¾ cups): Calories: 185; Total Fat: 0g; Saturated Fat: 0g; Trans Fat: 0g; Polyunsaturated Fat: 0g; Monounsaturated Fat: 0g; Cholesterol: 0mg; Sodium: 140mg; Carbohydrates: 34g; Fiber: 13g; Sugars: 6g; Protein: 11g

NUTRITIONAL HIGHLIGHT: Lentils are a very good source of cholesterol-lowering fiber. Not only do lentils help lower cholesterol, but the high fiber content keeps blood sugar levels steady for hours. The significant amounts of folate and magnesium in lentils also contribute to their heart-health benefits.

BARLEY AND CHICKPEA RISOTTO

Prep time: 10 minutes / Cook time: 6 to 7 hours on low

Traditional risotto is an Italian rice dish cooked in a broth to a creamy consistency. It is considered by most to be a complicated dish because you have to watch it carefully and stir constantly. This no-fuss recipe lets the slow cooker do the work for you by swapping rice for hulled barley, a slow-cooking grain with a chewy consistency. This meatless meal—creamy, filling, satisfying, and packed with protein—won't disappoint.

Serves 8

5 cups Savory Vegetable Broth (page 24) or low-sodium vegetable broth

2 cups hulled barley, rinsed

1 (15-ounce) can chickpeas, drained and rinsed

1 cup water

3 carrots, minced

1 onion, finely chopped

½ head cauliflower, cut into small pieces

4 garlic cloves, minced

1 teaspoon dried thyme

1½ tablespoons freshly squeezed lemon juice

⅓ cup grated Parmesan cheese

4 tablespoons chopped fresh parsley, for garnish (optional)

1. Put the broth, barley, chickpeas, water, carrots, onion, cauliflower, garlic, and thyme in a 6-quart slow cooker. Stir to combine. Cover and cook on low for 6 to 7 hours, or until the barley is tender and has absorbed most of the liquid.

2. Stir in the lemon juice and Parmesan cheese. Serve garnished with the fresh parsley (if using).

Per Serving (1½ cups): Calories: 267; Total Fat: 2g; Saturated Fat: 1g; Trans Fat: 0g; Polyunsaturated Fat: 0g; Monounsaturated Fat: 1g; Cholesterol: 2mg; Sodium: 183mg; Carbohydrates: 50g; Fiber: 13g; Sugars: 4g; Protein: 11g

COOKING TIP: Pearl barley is the most common form of barley. The outer husk and bran layers have been removed. Hulled barley is the whole-grain form of barley; it has only the outermost hull removed. Chewy and rich in fiber, it is the healthiest kind of barley and takes about twice as long to cook as pearl barley, making it ideal for the slow cooker.

VEGETARIAN CALICO BEANS

Prep time: 10 minutes, plus overnight to soak / Cook time: 7 to 8 hours on low

Beans are one of those heart-healthy staples that should be worked into your menu on a regular basis. This delicious calico bean recipe is high in protein, fiber, B vitamins, and minerals and can help lower cholesterol, as well as manage weight.

Serves 8

6 cups Savory Vegetable Broth (page 24) or low-sodium vegetable broth

1 (15-ounce) can lima beans, drained and rinsed

1 (14.5-ounce) can fire-roasted tomatoes

1 cup dried kidney beans, soaked overnight

1 cup dried pinto beans, soaked overnight

1 large sweet onion, chopped

1 medium red bell pepper, chopped

½ cup Homemade Ketchup (page 20)

⅓ cup loosely packed brown sugar

1 tablespoon Dijon mustard

1 tablespoon apple cider vinegar

Freshly ground black pepper

1. Combine the ingredients in a 6-quart slow cooker. Cover and cook on low for 7 to 8 hours, until the beans are tender.

2. Serve warm.

Per Serving (1⅓ cups): Calories: 246; Total Fat: 0g; Saturated Fat: 0g; Trans Fat: 0g; Polyunsaturated Fat: 0g; Monounsaturated Fat: 0g; Cholesterol: 0mg; Sodium: 331mg; Carbohydrates: 47g; Fiber: 9g; Sugars: 12g; Protein: 13g

COOKING TIP: You can swap out the dried beans in this recipe by replacing each cup with a 15-ounce can. Just be certain to drain and rinse the beans to remove excess sodium and reduce the cooking time to 5 to 6 hours.

SAVORY GREAT NORTHERN BEANS

Prep time: **10 minutes** / Cook time: **7 to 8 hours on low**

This recipe for great northern beans is very versatile, and you can easily change the seasonings or vegetables to match your preferred taste and depending on what you have on hand. A small white bean, great northerns are creamy and delicious and used in a diverse assortment of recipes such as crostini, minestrone soup, *pasta e fagioli*, and a side dish of bean stew with garlic and rosemary.

Serves 8

6 cups water

1 pound dried great
  northern beans

2 celery ribs, chopped

1 large onion, chopped

4 garlic cloves, minced

2 bay leaves

¼ teaspoon freshly ground
  black pepper

1. Rinse the beans well and pick them over. Discard any small stones you may find.

2. Combine all the ingredients in a 6-quart slow cooker and stir. Cover and cook on low for 7 to 8 hours, until the beans are tender.

3. Use the beans in any recipe calling for great northern beans. Freeze in airtight containers.

Per Serving (¾ cup): Calories: 206; Total Fat: 0g; Saturated Fat: 0g; Trans Fat: 0g; Polyunsaturated Fat: 0g; Monounsaturated Fat: 0g; Cholesterol: 0mg; Sodium: 15mg; Carbohydrates: 38g; Fiber: 12g; Sugars: 3g; Protein: 13g

COOKING TIP: Because great northern beans are small, it isn't necessary to soak them before cooking. However, if you find they did not become tender enough for you after so cooking, then go ahead and soak them overnight before making the recipe again.

CUBAN BLACK BEANS

Prep time: 10 minutes / Cook time: 6 to 7 hours on low

This recipe for black beans doesn't require presoaking to create a dish that is both authentic and delicious. The cumin and oregano give this recipe its traditional Cuban flavor, but if you want more of a recipe-ready bean preparation to use in other dishes, feel free to omit them.

Serves 8

1 pound dried black beans, picked over and rinsed

3 cups water

2 cups Savory Vegetable Broth (page 24) low-sodium vegetable broth

1 (14.5-ounce) can no-salt-added diced tomatoes

1 (4-ounce) can chopped green chiles (more or less to taste)

1 green bell pepper, chopped

1 large onion, chopped

6 garlic cloves, minced

2 bay leaves

1 teaspoon ground cumin

1 teaspoon dried oregano

Freshly ground black pepper

2 tablespoons freshly squeezed lime juice (optional)

1. Put the beans, water, broth, tomatoes, chiles, bell pepper, onion, garlic, bay leaves, cumin, oregano, and pepper in a 6-quart slow cooker. Stir to combine. Cover and cook on low for 6 to 7 hours, until the beans are tender.

2. Before serving, remove and discard the bay leaves. Stir in the lime juice (if using). Serve hot over rice.

Per Serving (1¼ cups): Calories: 224; Total Fat: 0g; Saturated Fat: 0g; Trans Fat: 0g; Polyunsaturated Fat: 0g; Monounsaturated Fat: 0g; Cholesterol: 0mg; Sodium: 78mg; Carbohydrates: 42g; Fiber: 13g; Sugars: 4g; Protein: 14g

COOKING TIP: This dish is traditionally served over rice, so no rice is added to the pot with the other ingredients. To save time, cook your rice the day before and simply reheat for serving with the beans.

MEDITERRANEAN BULGUR AND LENTILS

Prep time: 10 minutes / Cook time: 7 to 8 hours on low

This Mediterranean-inspired dish is thick, flavorful, nutritious, and full of satiating plant protein, fiber, and heart-healthy vitamins and minerals. Bulgur wheat is the main ingredient in many traditional Mediterranean meals, including tabbouleh. Enjoy this meal with olives and feta cheese. Add some fresh mint if you have it.

Serves 8

1 cup lentils

6 cups Savory Vegetable Broth (page 24) or Chicken Stock (page 25)

4 medium tomatoes, chopped with juices (about 3 cups)

2 cups bulgur wheat

1 large onion, chopped

4 garlic cloves, minced

1 teaspoon ground cumin

2 tablespoons pitted, chopped Kalamata olives

2 ounces crumbled reduced-fat feta cheese

Chopped fresh mint (optional)

1. Pick over the lentils, removing any debris, then rinse and drain well.

2. Put the broth, tomatoes, bulgur wheat, lentils, onion, garlic, and cumin in a 6-quart slow cooker. Stir well. Cover and cook on low for 7 to 8 hours, until the lentils and bulgur are tender.

3. Serve hot, garnished with the olives and feta cheese. Add fresh mint (if using).

Per Serving (1¼ cups): Calories: 217; Total Fat: 2g; Saturated Fat: 1g; Trans Fat: 0g; Polyunsaturated Fat: 1g; Monounsaturated Fat: 0g; Cholesterol: 2mg; Sodium: 265mg; Carbohydrates: 44g; Fiber: 14g; Sugars: 3g; Protein: 11g

INGREDIENT TIP: Olives are an excellent source of heart-healthy monounsaturated fats and make a nutritious addition to the diet. However, they are high in sodium, so keep portions in check.

RUSTIC HERBED MUSHROOM RICE

Prep time: 10 minutes / Cook time: 6 to 7 hours on low

This recipe for mushroom rice is simple yet elegant, with a rich, earthy taste from meaty mushrooms and rustic seasonings like garlic, rosemary, and thyme. Chickpeas are added to boost the protein and fiber content, making this a perfect side dish or main meal. Feel free to change up the types of mushrooms, herbs, and beans to make the recipe your own.

Serves 8

4 cups Beef Stock (page 27) or low-sodium beef broth

2 cups water

2 cups long-grain brown rice

1 (15-ounce) can chickpeas, drained and rinsed

1 cup sliced button mushrooms

1 cup sliced baby portobello mushrooms

½ cup dried shiitake mushrooms

¼ cup dry cooking sherry

4 garlic cloves, minced

1 tablespoon extra-virgin olive oil

1 teaspoon dried thyme

1 teaspoon dried rosemary

Freshly ground black pepper

1. Combine all the ingredients in a 6-quart slow cooker. Cover and cook on low for 6 to 7 hours, until the rice is tender.

2. Serve hot.

Per Serving (¾ cup): Calories: 250; Total Fat: 3g; Saturated Fat: 0g; Trans Fat: 0g; Polyunsaturated Fat: 0g; Monounsaturated Fat: 1g; Cholesterol: 0mg; Sodium: 221mg; Carbohydrates: 53g; Fiber: 5g; Sugars: 1g; Protein: 9g

NUTRITIONAL HIGHLIGHT: Wild mushrooms are one of the few foods rich in vitamin D, a nutrient many Americans are lacking. This meaty vegetable is also a leading source of the antioxidant selenium and rich in B vitamins and minerals.

FARRO AND PEA RISOTTO

Prep time: 10 minutes / Cook time: 6 to 7 hours on low

Farro is an ancient grain that has been around for thousands of years but has recently become popular. Not only does it taste great with its chewy texture, it's also really good for your health. This nutritious grain, full of fiber, protein, vitamins, minerals, and antioxidants, is used in this risotto-type dish with green peas and meaty mushrooms.

Serves 8

5 cups Savory Vegetable Broth (page 24) or low-sodium vegetable broth

2 cups whole farro

2 cups frozen peas

1 cup sliced button mushrooms

1 large leek, white and light green parts only, halved and thinly sliced

4 garlic cloves, minced

1 tablespoon extra-virgin olive oil

Freshly ground black pepper

⅓ cup grated Parmesan cheese

½ cup fresh parsley, chopped

1. Put the broth, farro, peas, mushrooms, leek, garlic, olive oil, and pepper in a 6-quart slow cooker and stir to combine. Cover and cook on low for 6 to 7 hours, until the farro and vegetables are tender.

2. Before serving, stir in the Parmesan cheese. Serve hot topped with the fresh parsley.

Per Serving (1⅛ cups): Calories: 241; Total Fat: 3g; Saturated Fat: 1g; Trans Fat: 0g; Polyunsaturated Fat: 0g; Monounsaturated Fat: 1g; Cholesterol: 4mg; Sodium: 227mg; Carbohydrates: 42g; Fiber: 5g; Sugars: 4g; Protein: 11g

COOKING TIP: Farro comes in whole-grain, pearled (perlato), and semi-pearled varieties. For maximum nutrition choose whole-grain farro as it contains the most fiber and protein.

INGREDIENT TIP: Farro contains gluten and is not suitable for people with celiac disease.

LEMON-SCENTED RISOTTO

Prep time: 10 minutes / Cook time: 5½ to 6½ hours on low

Using the slow cooker to make risotto is a great timesaver and a way for you to enjoy the signature creaminess of this dish more often—but without the intensive labor it takes to make traditional risotto. This version includes the bright taste of lemon!

Serves 8

5 cups Chicken Stock (page 25) or low-sodium chicken broth

2 cups short-grain brown rice

1 cup water

4 garlic cloves, minced

4 shallots, minced

1 tablespoon extra-virgin olive oil

1 teaspoon dried thyme

½ cup fresh grated Parmesan cheese

2 teaspoons lemon zest

1 tablespoon freshly squeezed lemon juice

Freshly ground black pepper

1. Put the stock, rice, water, garlic, shallots, olive oil, and thyme in a 6-quart slow cooker. Stir well. Cover and cook on low for 5 to 6 hours, until the rice is tender.

2. Stir in the Parmesan cheese, lemon zest, and lemon juice and continue cooking on low for 20 minutes more. Season with the pepper.

3. Serve hot.

Per Serving (⅔ cup): Calories: 224; Total Fat: 5g; Saturated Fat: 1g; Trans Fat: 0g; Polyunsaturated Fat: 0g; Monounsaturated Fat: 1g; Cholesterol: 6mg; Sodium: 239mg; Carbohydrates: 41g; Fiber: 3g; Sugars: 0g; Protein: 7g

SUBSTITUTION TIP: If you need to make this recipe dairy-free, there are a number of delicious vegan Parmesan cheese options. One brand to look for is Follow Your Heart. You could also substitute nutritional yeast for the cheese.

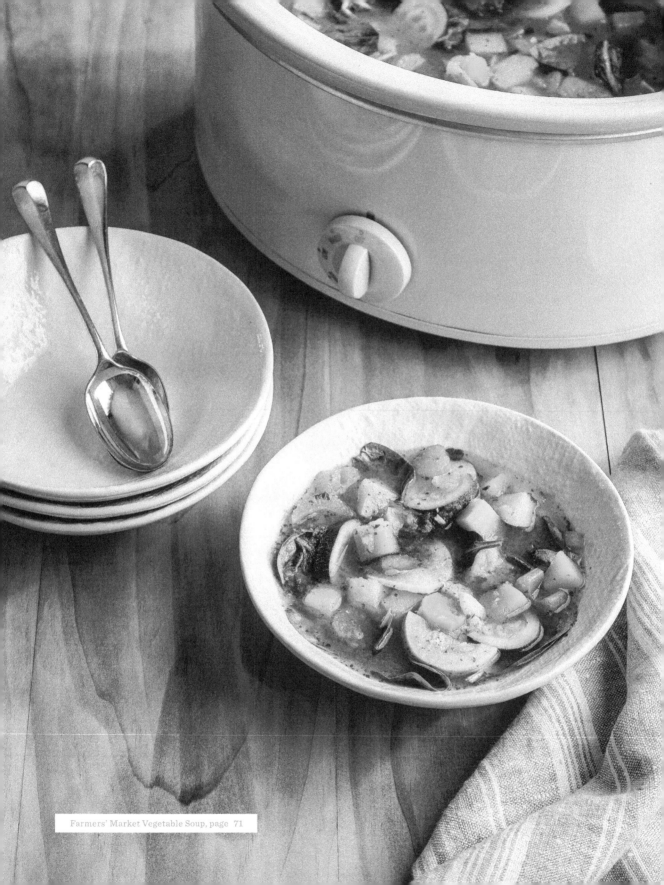

Farmers' Market Vegetable Soup, page 71

5

Soups, Stews, and Curries

POTATO AND CORN CHOWDER

Prep time: 10 minutes / Cook time: 7 to 8 hours on low

Nothing says comfort food better than a hot bowl of homemade potato and corn chowder. This fiber-rich soup is creamy and delicious and quick to put together with just a few pantry staples. Comfort food like this is heart-healthy, too. It's the best of both worlds!

Serves 8

1½ pounds red potatoes, diced

1 (16-ounce) package frozen corn

2 medium carrots, chopped

1 large onion, chopped

3 tablespoons all-purpose flour

5 cups Savory Vegetable Broth (page 24) or low-sodium vegetable broth

2 teaspoons dried thyme

4 garlic cloves, minced

1 tablespoon extra-virgin olive oil

Salt

Freshly ground black pepper

1 (12-ounce) can evaporated nonfat milk

1. Place the potatoes, corn, carrots, and onion into a 6-quart slow cooker. Stir in the flour and gently toss to combine. Stir in the broth, thyme, garlic, and olive oil. Season with salt and pepper.

2. Cover and cook on low for 7 to 8 hours. Thirty minutes before serving, stir in the evaporated milk and continue cooking until heated through.

3. Serve immediately.

Per Serving (1¾ cups): Calories: 208; Total Fat: 2g; Saturated Fat: 0g; Trans Fat: 0g; Polyunsaturated Fat: 1g; Monounsaturated Fat: 1g; Cholesterol: 2mg; Sodium: 172mg; Carbohydrates: 41g; Fiber: 4g; Sugars: 11g; Protein: 8g

COOKING TIP: Almost any type of potato will work in this recipe depending on the texture you prefer. Red potatoes hold their shape a bit better, but russet potatoes will make for a thicker soup.

AFRICAN PEANUT STEW

Prep time: 10 minutes / Cook time: 7 to 8 hours on low

If you have never tried a savory peanut dish before, you are in for a treat. Not only does the peanut butter create rich flavor in this stew, it thickens the sauce deliciously. Prep this in the morning and come home to the warm aroma of African-inspired food full of lean high-quality protein, fiber, and nutrient-rich veggies.

Serves 6 to 8

4 cups Chicken Stock (page 25) or low-sodium chicken broth

1 (14.5-ounce) can no-salt-added diced tomatoes

½ cup chunky peanut butter

1 tablespoon ground cumin

1 teaspoon ground coriander

¼ teaspoon salt

3 tablespoons minced fresh ginger

2 pounds boneless, skinless chicken breasts, cut into 1-inch pieces

1 large sweet potato (about 1 pound), peeled and cubed

2 medium zucchini (1 pound), cubed

1 (14.5-ounce) can chickpeas, drained and rinsed

½ cup chopped roasted unsalted peanuts

¼ cup chopped cilantro

1. In a blender or food processor, add the stock, tomatoes, peanut butter, cumin, coriander, and salt and blend until thick and pasty.

2. In a 6-quart slow cooker, combine the ginger, chicken, sweet potato, zucchini, and chickpeas. Pour the sauce over the chicken and vegetables. Cover and cook on low for 7 to 8 hours. The finished stew should reach a temperature of 165°F.

3. Garnish the finished stew with the chopped peanuts and cilantro.

Per Serving (1½ cups): Calories: 476; Total Fat: 21g; Saturated Fat: 5g; Trans Fat: 0g; Polyunsaturated Fat: 5g; Monounsaturated Fat: 10g; Cholesterol: 87mg; Sodium: 345mg; Carbohydrates: 28g; Fiber: 7g; Sugars: 8g; Protein: 47g

NUTRITIONAL HIGHLIGHT: Eating nuts as part of a healthy diet is good for your heart. Nuts contain unsaturated, healthy fatty acids and other nutrients. They are a great snack food, inexpensive, and easy to grab and go. Aim for 1 to 1½ ounces per day.

LEMON CHICKEN ORZO SOUP

Prep time: **15 minutes** / Cook time: **7 to 8 hours on low**

This family-friendly, bright-tasting lemon chicken orzo soup is full of heart-healthy nutrients, simple to prep and make, and super satisfying. The parsley and lemon juice perk up the taste to take this recipe beyond the usual chicken soup.

Serves 6

1 pound boneless, skinless chicken breasts

4 cups Savory Vegetable Broth (page 24) or low-sodium vegetable broth

2 cups Chicken Stock (page 25) or low-sodium chicken broth

2 large carrots, sliced

2 celery stalks, finely chopped

6 garlic cloves, minced

1 teaspoon dried basil

1 teaspoon Italian seasoning

2 bay leaves

Juice of 1 lemon

½ cup chopped fresh parsley

8 ounces orzo (whole-wheat is ideal)

Freshly ground black pepper

1. Place the chicken, vegetable broth, chicken stock, carrots, celery, garlic, basil, Italian seasoning, and bay leaves in a 6-quart slow cooker. Cover and cook on low for 7 to 8 hours.

2. About 30 minutes prior to serving, remove discard the bay leaves. Use two forks to shred the chicken. Stir in the lemon juice, parsley, orzo, and pepper. Cook for 30 minutes, until the orzo is tender, stirring every 10 minutes or so because the orzo may stick to the bottom of the slow cooker.

3. Serve immediately.

Per Serving (1⅔ cups): Calories: 259; Total Fat: 2g; Saturated Fat: 1g; Trans Fat: 0g; Polyunsaturated Fat: 1g; Monounsaturated Fat: 1g; Cholesterol: 43mg; Sodium: 179mg; Carbohydrates: 34g; Fiber: 3g; Sugars: 3g; Protein: 25g

SUBSTITUTION TIP: You can make this recipe gluten-free by using quinoa or brown rice in place of the orzo.

BUTTERNUT SQUASH CHILI

Prep time: 10 minutes / Cook time: 7 to 8 hours on low

This spicy, flavorful chili is packed with satiating plant protein, energy-sustaining complex carbohydrates, healthy vitamins, minerals, phytonutrients, and fiber to create a heart-healthy nutrient-dense meal.

Serves 6 to 8

6 cups Savory Vegetable Broth (page 24), low-sodium vegetable broth, or water

4 cups cubed butternut squash

2 (14.5-ounce) cans cannellini beans, drained and rinsed

1 (14.5-ounce) can no-salt-added fire-roasted tomatoes

1 cup quinoa, well rinsed

1 large white or yellow onion, diced

1 red bell pepper, diced

4 garlic cloves, minced

2 teaspoons chili powder

1 teaspoon ground cumin

½ teaspoon smoked paprika

½ teaspoon ground cinnamon

Pinch salt

1. Combine all of the ingredients in a 6-quart slow cooker. Cover and cook on low for 7 to 8 hours.

2. Serve warm.

Per Serving (2 cups): Calories: 323; Total Fat: 2g; Saturated Fat: 0g; Trans Fat: 0g; Polyunsaturated Fat: 1g; Monounsaturated Fat: 1g; Cholesterol: 0mg; Sodium: 101mg; Carbohydrates: 65g; Fiber: 14g; Sugars: 11g; Protein: 15g

COOKING TIP: Although you can buy a whole butternut squash and do the peeling and cubing yourself, you can save time and spend about the same amount of money by purchasing a package of fresh peeled and cubed squash. Look for it in the produce section of your grocery store.

YELLOW DAL CURRY

Prep time: 10 minutes / Cook time: 7 to 8 hours on low

Flavorful and fragrant, tasty and filling, dal makes a nutritious, healthy, inexpensive, and satisfying meal. It has a hearty foundation of tender yellow split peas and the aroma of Indian spices will greet you when you open the lid of the slow cooker.

Serves 6 to 8

2 cups dried yellow split peas or lentils, rinsed

5 cups Savory Vegetable Broth (page 24), or low-sodium vegetable broth

1 (14.5-ounce) can no-salt-added crushed tomatoes

1 onion, diced

4 garlic cloves, minced

2 tablespoons finely chopped fresh ginger

1 tablespoon curry powder

1 teaspoon ground cumin

1 teaspoon ground coriander

1 teaspoon ground turmeric

Freshly ground black pepper

1. Combine all the ingredients in a 6-quart slow cooker. Cover and cook on low for 7 to 8 hours until thickened.

2. Serve warm over hot rice, if desired.

Per Serving (1½ cups): Calories: 185; Total Fat: 0g; Saturated Fat: 0g; Trans Fat: 0g; Polyunsaturated Fat: 0g; Monounsaturated Fat: 0g; Cholesterol: 0mg; Sodium: 157mg; Carbohydrates: 44g; Fiber: 17g; Sugars: 6g; Protein: 16g

VARIATION TIP: For additional fiber, vitamins, and minerals, stir in 5 ounces of baby spinach during the last 5 minutes of cooking.

CREAMY SWEET POTATO SOUP

Prep time: 15 minutes / Cook time: 7 to 8 hours on low

This velvety and savory sweet potato soup is rich in vitamins and minerals, and the touch of spice from the minced fresh ginger makes it so aromatic. Enjoy this nourishing vegan and gluten-free soup garnished with some roasted (unsalted) pumpkin seeds on top.

Serves 6

4 medium sweet potatoes, sliced

4 cups Savory Vegetable Broth (page 24) or low-sodium vegetable broth

2 cups unsweetened almond milk or low-fat milk

2 medium carrots, chopped

1 onion, sliced

1 tablespoon minced garlic

1 tablespoon minced fresh ginger

2 teaspoons ground cumin

⅛ teaspoon ground nutmeg

Freshly ground black pepper

1. Combine all the ingredients in a 6-quart slow cooker. Cover and cook on low for 7 to 8 hours.

2. Using an immersion blender or standing blender, blend the soup until smooth.

3. Serve warm.

Per Serving (1½ cups): 124; Total Fat: 0g; Saturated Fat: 0g; Trans Fat: 0g; Polyunsaturated Fat: 0g; Monounsaturated Fat: 0g; Cholesterol: 0mg; Sodium: 192mg; Carbohydrates: 27g; Fiber: 5g; Sugars: 20g; Protein: 2g

NUTRITIONAL HIGHLIGHT: Sweet potatoes are an excellent source of vitamin A (in the form of beta-carotene), and a good source of fiber, B vitamins, vitamin C, and the heart-healthy blood pressure–regulating mineral potassium.

MINESTRONE SOUP

Prep time: 15 minutes / Cook time: 7 to 8 hours on low

Slow cooking this crowd-pleasing soup allows the flavors to intensify and develop for a meal the whole family is sure to enjoy. This hearty and tasty version with a thick rich tomato sauce uses barley in place of elbow pasta to take advantage of barley's cholesterol-lowering properties. Serve with a green salad and crusty whole-grain bread.

Serves 6 to 8

6 cups Savory Vegetable Broth (page 24) or low-sodium vegetable broth

1 (28-ounce) can no-salt-added diced tomatoes

1 (14.5-ounce) can white kidney beans, drained and rinsed

1 (14.5-ounce) can red kidney beans, drained and rinsed

2 large onions, chopped

3 celery stalks, chopped

2 carrots, chopped

1 medium zucchini, diced

1½ cups fresh green beans, trimmed and cut into ½-inch pieces

1 cup chopped fresh spinach

½ cup hulled barley

4 garlic cloves, minced

1 tablespoon chopped fresh parsley

Freshly ground black pepper

1. Combine all the ingredients in a 6-quart slow cooker. Cover and cook on low for 7 to 8 hours.

2. Serve warm.

Per Serving (2 cups): Calories: 254; Total Fat: 0g; Saturated Fat: 0g; Trans Fat: 0g; Polyunsaturated Fat: 0g; Monounsaturated Fat: 0g; Cholesterol: 0mg; Sodium: 188mg; Carbohydrates: 52g; Fiber: 13g; Sugars: 11g; Protein: 12g

VARIATION TIP: If you prefer a more traditional minestrone and have time to tend to the slow cooker toward the end of cooking, skip the barley and add in 1 cup of your preferred pasta 30 to 40 minutes before the soup is done and cook until the pasta is tender. The pasta will need to be stirred occasionally while it cooks to prevent it from sticking to the bottom of the slow cooker.

FARMERS' MARKET VEGETABLE SOUP

Prep time: 15 minutes / Cook time: 7 to 8 hours on low

Many slow cooker recipes call for throwing random ingredients into the pot and hoping for something delicious. But this soup has that something extra that elevates it beyond the ordinary. While the stars are certainly the fiber- and nutrient-rich vegetables, the addition of the onion and garlic purée takes it to another level, resulting in a soup that is deeply flavorful and quite delicious.

Serves 6 to 8

4 medium potatoes such as Yukon gold, cut into 1-inch cubes

2 cups peeled and cubed butternut squash (about 1½ pounds)

2 small yellow squash or zucchini, sliced

4 celery stalks, chopped

3 large carrots, chopped

1 medium onion, chopped

4 garlic cloves, peeled

¼ cup packed fresh cilantro

¼ cup packed fresh basil leaves

2 tablespoons extra-virgin olive oil

6 cups Savory Vegetable Broth (page 24) or low-sodium vegetable broth

⅛ teaspoon salt

Freshly ground black pepper

4 cups baby spinach

Juice of ½ lemon

1. Put the potatoes, butternut squash, yellow squash, celery, and carrots in a 6-quart slow cooker.

2. Place the onion, garlic, cilantro, basil, and olive oil into a food processor. Blend until it achieves a coarse and chunky consistency. Pour this into the slow cooker.

3. Next add the broth, salt, and pepper and stir to combine. Cover and cook on low for 7 to 8 hours.

4. Stir in the spinach and lemon juice about 30 minutes before serving.

5. Serve warm.

Per Serving (2 cups): Calories: 200; Total Fat: 5g; Saturated Fat: 1g; Trans Fat: 0g; Polyunsaturated Fat: 1g; Monounsaturated Fat: 3g; Cholesterol: 0mg; Sodium: 256mg; Carbohydrates: 37g; Fiber: 8g; Sugars: 8g; Protein: 5g

NUTRITIONAL HIGHLIGHT: Olive oil is rich in heart-healthy monounsaturated fatty acids and powerful antioxidants that protect against heart disease, type 2 diabetes, and some types of cancer; reduce inflammation; and may help with weight management as part of a heart-healthy diet.

CHICKEN TORTILLA SOUP

Prep time: 15 minutes / Cook time: 7 to 8 hours on low

With 15 minutes of prep time, this slow cooker chicken tortilla soup is incredibly flavorful and hearty; it's perfect for chilly days. Loaded with healthy ingredients, including ample amounts of protein from the chicken and fiber-rich beans, this soup will keep you full and satisfied. It's a true recipe staple to have in your back pocket.

Serves 6 to 8

1½ pounds boneless, skinless chicken breasts

6 cups Chicken Stock (page 25) or low-sodium chicken broth

1 (14.5-ounce) can black beans, drained and rinsed

1 (14.5-ounce) can whole kernel corn, drained and rinsed

1 (14.5-ounce) can no-salt-added diced fire-roasted tomatoes

3 garlic cloves, minced

1 medium onion, finely chopped

2 bell peppers (any color), chopped

1 tablespoon chili powder

2 teaspoons ground cumin

¾ teaspoon smoked paprika

¼ cup freshly squeezed lime juice

Optional toppings: tortilla strips or chips, diced or sliced avocado, diced fresh tomatoes, shredded cheese, chopped cilantro, or sour cream

1. Put the chicken, stock, black beans, corn, tomatoes, garlic, onion, bell peppers, chili powder, cumin, and paprika in a 6-quart slow cooker and stir to combine. Cover and cook on low for 7 to 8 hours, until chicken is tender and cooked through.

2. Remove chicken and use two forks to shred it. Return chicken to the slow cooker and stir in the lime juice. Cook until the chicken is heated through again.

3. Serve warm with toppings such as tortilla strips or chips, diced or sliced avocado, diced fresh tomatoes, shredded cheese, chopped cilantro, or sour cream, if desired.

Per Serving (2 cups): Calories: 290; Total Fat: 4g; Saturated Fat: 1g; Trans Fat: 0g; Polyunsaturated Fat: 1g; Monounsaturated Fat: 2g; Cholesterol: 65mg; Sodium: 145mg; Carbohydrates: 32g; Fiber: 6g; Sugars: 8g; Protein: 33g

VARIATION TIP: When choosing toppings for the most heart-healthy benefits, opt for low-fat plain Greek yogurt in place of sour cream. With similar consistencies and flavor, making this swap will cut down on unhealthy fats while boosting the calcium and protein content.

SQUASH AND LENTIL STEW

Prep time: 10 minutes / Cook time: 7 to 8 hours on low

This stew contains all types of wonderful ingredients: big chunks of winter squash, spicy bits of jalapeño peppers, red lentils, tomatoes, and carrots. Seasoned with fragrant herbs and spices, this stew is truly a vegan treat.

Serves 6 to 8

6 cups Savory Vegetable Broth (page 24) or low-sodium vegetable broth

3 pounds kabocha squash or butternut squash, peeled, seeded, and cut into 1-inch cubes (about 4 to 4½ cups)

1 (28-ounce) can no-salt-added diced tomatoes

1 cup red lentils

2 large carrots, cut into ½-inch pieces

1 large onion, chopped

1 jalapeño pepper, seeded and minced

3 garlic cloves, minced

1 tablespoon garam masala

Freshly ground black pepper

1. Put the broth, squash, chickpeas, tomatoes, lentils, carrots, onion, jalapeño, garlic, garam masala, and pepper in a 6-quart slow cooker and stir to combine. Cover and cook on low for 7 to 8 hours: The longer you cook it, the thicker your stew will be.

2. Serve warm garnished with the cilantro.

Per Serving (1¾ cups): Calories: 364; Total Fat: 0g; Saturated Fat: 0g; Trans Fat: 0g; Polyunsaturated Fat: 0g; Monounsaturated Fat: 0g; Cholesterol: 0mg; Sodium: 179mg; Carbohydrates: 71g; Fiber: 20g; Sugars: 14g; Protein: 19g

VARIATION TIP: If you have the time, you can enhance the flavor of this stew by heating 1 tablespoon of extra-virgin olive oil in a large skillet over medium-high heat. Add the onion, carrots, and jalapeño and sauté until the onion is translucent, about 6 minutes.. Add the minced garlic and garam masala, stirring well to coat. Add this to the slow cooker with the rest of the ingredients, cover, and cook.

MIDDLE EASTERN LAMB STEW

Prep time: 10 minutes / Cook time: 7 to 8 hours on low

This boldly flavored Middle Eastern lamb stew is full of fiber-rich chickpeas and lamb that tenderizes beautifully when cooked for hours in the slow cooker. Serve this rich, brothy, and fragrant stew over whole-wheat couscous for a traditional Middle Eastern comfort meal.

Serves 8

2 pounds boneless lamb stew meat, cut into 1-inch chunks, or 2½ pounds lamb shoulder chops, deboned and trimmed

1 (28-ounce) can no-salt-added diced tomatoes

1 (14.5-ounce) can chickpeas, drained and rinsed

¾ cup Beef Stock (page 27) or low-sodium beef broth

1 large onion, chopped

2 garlic cloves, minced

2 teaspoons grated fresh ginger

2 teaspoons ground cumin

½ teaspoon ground cinnamon

½ teaspoon dried mint

¼ teaspoon freshly ground black pepper

1 tablespoon freshly squeezed lemon juice

Pinch salt

1. Place the lamb in a 6-quart slow cooker. Add the tomatoes, chickpeas, stock, onion, garlic, ginger, cumin, cinnamon, mint, and pepper and stir well. Cover and cook on low for 7 to 8 hours.

2. Turn off the slow cooker and stir in the lemon juice and salt. Let the stew stand for 5 minutes to allow the flavors to blend. Serve warm.

Per Serving (1 cup): Calories: 251; Total Fat: 9g; Saturated Fat: 4g; Trans Fat: 0g; Polyunsaturated Fat: 2g; Monounsaturated Fat: 3g; Cholesterol: 55mg; Sodium: 164mg; Carbohydrates: 18g; Fiber: 4g; Sugars: 6g; Protein: 27g

MAKE-AHEAD: You can mix the ingredients, cover, and refrigerate for up to 2 days prior to cooking.

APPLE-PARSNIP SOUP

Prep time: 10 minutes / Cook time: 7 to 8 hours on low

Parsnips are one of those underrated vegetables that people commonly miss in the grocery store. However, this humble vegetable is delicious and versatile and contains high levels of heart-healthy potassium, vitamins, minerals, and fiber. With added sweetness from apples and a touch of heat from curry powder, this creamy soup is hearty and sure to please.

Serves 6 to 8

6 parsnips (about 2 pounds), peeled and cut into chunks

5 large Granny Smith apples, peeled, cored, and quartered

4 cups Savory Vegetable Broth (page 24)

4 cups water

1 (15-ounce) can cannellini beans, drained and rinsed, or 1½ to 2 cups Savory Great Northern Beans (page 56)

1 Vidalia onion, finely chopped

1 large red bell pepper, chopped

6 garlic cloves, minced

1 tablespoon curry powder

Freshly ground black pepper

Extra-virgin olive oil, for garnish

1. Add the parsnips, apples, broth, water, beans, onion, bell pepper, garlic, curry powder, and pepper to a 6-quart slow cooker and stir to combine. Cover and cook on low for 7 to 8 hours, until the parsnips are tender.

2. Using an immersion blender, purée the soup until smooth.

3. Serve immediately with a drizzle of olive oil as a garnish, if desired.

Per Serving (1⅔ cups): Calories: 316; Total Fat: 1g; Saturated Fat: 0g; Trans Fat: 0g; Polyunsaturated Fat: 0g; Monounsaturated Fat: 0g; Cholesterol: 0mg; Sodium: 112mg; Carbohydrates: 67g; Fiber: 17g; Sugars: 27g; Protein: 8g

VARIATION TIP: You can replace the beans with 1½ cups red lentils for a curry soup that's more traditional in both taste and color.

ROOT VEGETABLE STEW

Prep time: 15 minutes / Cook time: 6 to 8 hours on low

Slow cooking root vegetables brings out their natural sweetness and can transform them into a delicious bowl of hearty and filling nourishment. This recipe is easy to customize with your favorite root vegetables and spices. You prep the vegetables and then your slow cooker does the rest!

Serves 6 to 8

1 pound Yukon gold
  potatoes, diced

1 pound sweet potatoes, diced

1 pound parsnips, diced

1 pound carrots, diced

4 cups Savory Vegetable
  Broth (page 24)

3 cups diced butternut squash

2 medium beets, peeled
  and diced

2 medium onions, diced

1 (15-ounce) can chickpeas,
  drained and rinsed

4 garlic cloves, minced

2 bay leaves

2 teaspoons dried sage

Freshly ground black pepper

1. Combine all the ingredients in a 6-quart slow cooker. Cover and cook on low for 6 to 8 hours, until the vegetables are tender.

2. Remove and discard the bay leaves and serve hot.

Per Serving (1½ cups): Calories: 357; Total Fat: 0g; Saturated Fat: 0g; Trans Fat: 0g; Polyunsaturated Fat: 0g; Monounsaturated Fat: 0g; Cholesterol: 0mg; Sodium: 240mg; Carbohydrates: 81g; Fiber: 16g; Sugars: 30g; Protein: 10g

COOKING TIP: If you prefer a thicker stew use, 3 cups of vegetable broth.

MAKE-AHEAD: Prep all of your vegetables the day before so that in the morning all you need to do is fill the slow cooker, turn it on, and go about your day.

CURRIED CARROT SOUP

Prep time: 10 minutes / Cook time: 7 to 8 hours on low

Soup is such a versatile meal option and a great way to boost your intake of nutritious vegetables. Plus the flavors of soups tend to intensify after a day or two, making them particularly delicious to eat throughout the week. With its creamy texture, ample vegetables, and flavorful curry taste, this soup makes a great meal or snack any time of the day.

Serves 6

4 cups Savory Vegetable Broth (page 24) or low-sodium vegetable broth

1½ pounds carrots, chopped

1 large onion, chopped

1 medium apple, peeled and diced

4 garlic cloves, minced

2 teaspoons curry powder

2 cups low-fat or fat-free milk, or plant-based milk

Freshly ground black pepper

1. Put the broth, carrots, onion, apple, garlic, and curry powder in the slow cooker and stir to combine. Cover and cook on low for 7 to 8 hours, until the carrots are very tender.

2. Using an immersion blender, purée the soup until smooth.

3. Blend in the milk, using more or less depending on how thick you want your soup to be.

4. Season with the pepper and serve hot. The soup may be topped with a dollop of plain Greek yogurt and a sprinkle of sliced scallions.

Per Serving (1¼ cups): Calories: 121; Total Fat: 1g; Saturated Fat: 1g; Trans Fat: 0g; Polyunsaturated Fat: 0g; Monounsaturated Fat: 0g; Cholesterol: 5mg; Sodium: 213mg; Carbohydrates: 24g; Fiber: 5g; Sugars: 14g; Protein: 4g

VARIATION TIP: For a coconut curry soup, replace the milk with light coconut milk or a coconut milk beverage. Just note that doing so will change the nutrition facts.

CHINESE PORK AND VEGETABLE HOT POT

Prep time: 15 minutes / Cook time: 7 to 8 hours on low

This Chinese pork stew has all of the characteristic rich flavors of Chinese cooking with none of the fuss of cooking this recipe on the stove top. The pork shoulder becomes meltingly tender during the slow-cooking process and delivers a warming winter meal.

Serves 8

1 pound fingerling potatoes, diced

4 medium carrots, sliced

2 celery stalks, cut into 2-inch chunks

1 medium onion, chopped

4 garlic cloves, minced

2 tablespoons grated fresh ginger

4 tablespoons all-purpose flour, divided

2½ pounds boneless pork shoulder, trimmed and cut into 1½-inch chunks

2 teaspoons dried thyme

½ teaspoon allspice

Freshly ground black pepper

3 cups Chicken Stock (page 25) or low-sodium chicken broth

1 (14.5-ounce) can no-salt-added diced tomatoes

1. Put the potatoes, carrots, celery, onion, garlic, and ginger in a 6-quart slow cooker. Sprinkle with 2 tablespoons of flour and stir to coat the vegetables.

2. Season the pork with the thyme, allspice, and pepper and toss with the remaining 2 tablespoons of flour to coat. Place the pork over the vegetables in the slow cooker. Add the stock and tomatoes. Cover and cook on low for 7 to 8 hours, until the meat and vegetables are tender.

3. Serve hot.

Per Serving (1¼ cups): Calories: 402; Total Fat: 22g; Saturated Fat: 8g; Trans Fat: 0g; Polyunsaturated Fat: 3g; Monounsaturated Fat: 10g; Cholesterol: 95mg; Sodium: 313mg; Carbohydrates: 21g; Fiber: 3g; Sugars: 5g; Protein: 28g

SUBSTITUTION TIP: You can make this recipe gluten-free by substituting almond meal for the all-purpose flour.

COCONUT CURRY CHICKEN

Prep time: 15 minutes / Cook time: 7 to 8 hours on low

This slow cooker coconut chicken curry is made with easy-to-find ingredients such as sweet potatoes and light coconut milk, with a touch of raisins that plump up during the slow-cooking process. A simple-to-prep, hearty Asian dinner, this dish is delicious served over fragrant jasmine rice.

Serves 6 to 8

Nonstick cooking spray

2 pounds boneless, skinless chicken breasts, cut into 1-inch cubes

6 medium carrots, diced

2 cups cubed butternut squash

1 large onion, diced

1 large green bell pepper, chopped

2 cups Chicken Stock (page 25) or low-sodium chicken broth

1 (14-ounce) can light coconut milk

1 (5-ounce) can tomato paste

4 garlic cloves, minced

2 tablespoons curry powder (or to taste)

Freshly ground black pepper

Chopped cashews (optional)

Chopped fresh cilantro (optional)

1. Spray a 6-quart slow cooker with the cooking spray. Add the chicken, carrots, butternut squash, onion, and bell pepper to the slow cooker.

2. Place the stock, coconut milk, tomato paste, garlic, curry powder, and black pepper in a food processor and process until smooth. Pour the mixture over the chicken and vegetables and mix well. Cover and cook on low for 7 to 8 hours, until the chicken and vegetables are cooked through.

3. During the last 30 minutes of cooking, remove the chicken and use two forks to shred it. Return the chicken to the slow cooker for the remaining cooking time.

4. Serve over jasmine rice, if desired, garnished with chopped cashews and cilantro.

Per Serving (1 cup): Calories: 327; Total Fat: 9g; Saturated Fat: 5g; Trans Fat: 0g; Polyunsaturated Fat: 1g; Monounsaturated Fat: 3g; Cholesterol: 87mg; Sodium: 202mg; Carbohydrates: 24g; Fiber: 6g; Sugars: 8g; Protein: 38g

COOKING TIP: If you prefer a thicker curry, whisk together 2 tablespoons of cornstarch and 3 tablespoons of water and stir into the slow cooker about 30 minutes before serving.

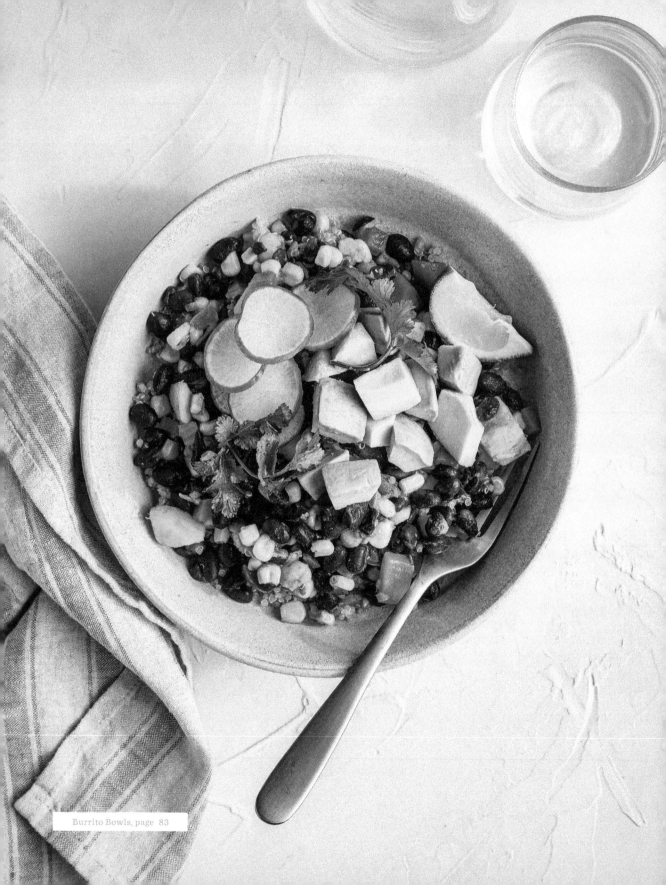

Burrito Bowls, page 83

6

Meatless Mains

VEGAN JAMBALAYA

Prep time: 15 minutes / Cook time: 6 to 8 hours on low

With traditional Cajun spices, this no-meat jambalaya is full of fiber-rich vegetables with a protein punch from the kidney beans. Cashews add healthy fats and a rich hearty flavor so you won't miss the meat.

Serves 6

5 cups Savory Vegetable Broth (page 24) or low-sodium vegetable broth

1 (15-ounce) can red kidney beans, drained and rinsed

2 cups diced fresh tomatoes with their juices, or 1 (14.5-ounce) can no-salt-added diced tomatoes

2 cups long-grain brown rice

1 cup ½-inch round okra slices

1 cup chopped cashews

2 celery stalks, diced

1 green bell pepper, diced

1 medium onion, diced

4 garlic cloves, minced

2 tablespoons cayenne hot sauce (or to taste)

1 tablespoon extra-virgin olive oil

1 tablespoon smoked paprika

1 tablespoon ground cumin

1 teaspoon dried thyme

1 teaspoon dried oregano

1. Combine all the ingredients in a 6-quart slow cooker. Cover and cook on low for 6 to 8 hours, until the vegetables and rice are tender and the sauce has thickened. If the rice becomes too dry during cooking, add more broth or water.

2. Serve hot.

Per Serving (1¾ cups): Calories: 504; Total Fat: 16g; Saturated Fat: 3g; Trans Fat: 0g; Polyunsaturated Fat: 2g; Monounsaturated Fat: 7g; Cholesterol: 0mg; Sodium: 153mg; Carbohydrates: 80g; Fiber: 9g; Sugars: 7g; Protein: 15g

SUBSTITUTION TIP: If gluten isn't a concern and you like the taste, add 1 to 2 cups of cooked vegan chorizo, seitan, or vegan sausage to the jambalaya before you serve it.

BURRITO BOWLS

Prep time: 15 minutes / Cook time: 7 to 8 hours on low

This recipe for burrito bowls just may become your new favorite go-to meal. Easy, quick, and delicious, there's no need to precook ingredients, plus it is easy to customize with whatever veggies and beans you have on hand.

Serves 6

2 (15-ounce) cans black
  beans, drained and rinsed

2 cups cubed sweet potato

1 (14.5-ounce) can no-salt-
  added diced tomatoes

1 cup Savory Vegetable
  Broth (page 24) or low-
  sodium vegetable broth

1 cup chopped onion

1 bell pepper, chopped

½ cup frozen corn

½ cup Spicy Salsa (page 19)

1 tablespoon hot sauce
  (or to taste)

1 teaspoon smoked paprika

½ teaspoon ground cumin

Freshly ground black pepper

Sliced avocado, radish,
  cilantro, and/or lime, for
  garnish (optional)

1. Combine all the ingredients in a 6-quart slow cooker. Cover and cook on low for 7 to 8 hours, until the vegetables are tender.

2. Serve hot with your favorite toppings.

Per Serving (1¾ cups): Calories: 192; Total Fat: 0g; Saturated Fat: 0g; Trans Fat: 0g; Polyunsaturated Fat: 0g; Monounsaturated Fat: 0g; Cholesterol: 0mg; Sodium: 121mg; Carbohydrates: 39g; Fiber: 8g; Sugars: 5g; Protein: 9g

VARIATION TIP: You can serve these burrito bowls simply with a green salad and toppings, you can use the bean-and-vegetable mixture as a filling for flour tortillas, or you can serve over your favorite grain.

LENTIL SHEPHERD'S PIE

Prep time: 10 minutes / Cook time: 6 to 7 hours on low

There are countless versions of shepherd's pie because it's one of those recipes that you can tweak to your liking. This version uses French lentilles du Puy, which hold up during the slow-cooking process, along with a mix of traditional shepherd's pie vegetables and seasonings, and is topped with a less-traditional mashed sweet potato topping. This is an easy and nourishing protein- and fiber-rich meal that is comfort food at its finest.

Serves 6

Nonstick cooking spray

3 cups Savory Vegetable Broth (page 24) or low-sodium vegetable broth

2 cups lentilles du Puy, picked over and rinsed well

1 (14.5-ounce) can no-salt-added diced tomatoes

1 large onion, diced

1 cup chopped mushrooms

4 celery stalks, diced

3 large carrots, diced

4 garlic cloves, crushed

1 tablespoon extra-virgin olive oil

1 teaspoon dried sage

½ teaspoon dried thyme

1 cup frozen peas

4 cups Perfect Sweet Potatoes (page 143), mashed

1. Spray the inside of a 6-quart slow cooker with cooking spray. Add the broth, lentils du Puy, tomatoes, onion, mushrooms, celery, carrots, garlic, olive oil, sage, and thyme and stir to combine. Cover and cook on low for 6 to 7 hours.

2. When the cooking time is complete, stir in the frozen peas.

3. Warm the mashed sweet potato in a microwave-safe dish until hot while the peas heat through.

4. To serve, spoon the shepherd's pie into bowls and top with a scoop of mashed sweet potatoes.

Per Serving (1¾ cups lentil mixture topped with ⅔ cup mashed sweet potatoes): Calories: 386; Total Fat: 3g; Saturated Fat: 0g; Trans Fat: 0g; Polyunsaturated Fat: 1g; Monounsaturated Fat: 2g; Cholesterol: 0mg; Sodium: 254mg; Carbohydrates: 72g; Fiber: 14g; Sugars: 14g; Protein: 18g

MAKE-AHEAD: Cook and mash the potatoes the day before and refrigerate them until you are ready to serve. For a more traditional version of shepherd's pie, you can use regular white potatoes instead of the sweet.

BLACK BEAN ENCHILADAS

Prep time: 15 minutes / Cook time: 6 to 8 hours on low

These easy slow cooker black bean enchiladas boast a heart-healthy vegetarian filling with no precooking required. Black beans, corn, tomatoes, peppers, onions, and Mexican spices are layered between corn tortillas and topped with salsa and cheese. Just prep it and come home to the aroma of fresh and hot homemade enchiladas.

Serves 6

2 (14.5-ounce) cans black beans, drained and rinsed

1 (14.5-ounce) can fire-roasted tomatoes with garlic drained and juice reserved

1 cup frozen corn kernels

1 bell pepper (any color), chopped

1 onion, chopped

1 (4-ounce) can green chiles

1 cup low-fat shredded Mexican cheese blend, divided

2 teaspoons ground cumin

Nonstick cooking spray

2 cups Spicy Salsa (page 19), divided

12 (6-inch) corn tortillas

1. In a large mixing bowl, mash the beans gently with a fork. Add the tomatoes, corn, bell pepper, onion, chiles, ½ cup of cheese, and cumin to the bowl and stir to combine.

2. Spray the inside of a 6-quart slow cooker with the cooking spray. Spread about 1 cup of salsa in the slow cooker, enough to evenly coat the bottom.

3. Dividing evenly, fill each tortilla with ½ cup of the bean filling, roll them up tight, and pack 6 of them seam-side down in a single layer in the bottom of the slow cooker. Spread ½ cup of salsa over the top and sprinkle with ¼ cup of cheese. Pack the remaining 6 enchiladas seam-side down to create a second layer. Finish by spreading the remaining ½ cup of salsa (and any remaining salsa juice) and ¼ cup of cheese on top.

4. Cover and cook on low for 6 to 8 hours.

5. Serve hot, with your favorite toppings.

Per Serving (2 enchiladas): Calories: 306; Total Fat: 4g; Saturated Fat: 2g; Trans Fat: 0g; Polyunsaturated Fat: 1g; Monounsaturated Fat: 1g; Cholesterol: 10mg; Sodium: 348mg; Carbohydrates: 50g; Fiber: 10g; Sugars: 12g; Protein: 15g

SUBSTITUTION TIP: You could use flour tortillas if you have them on hand, but they tend to get soggy when they soak up the salsa and cooking juices. Note that using flour tortillas will remove this recipe from the gluten-free category.

STUFFED SHELLS

Prep time: 15 minutes / Cook time: 6 to 8 hours on low

These slow cooker stuffed shells get a nutrition boost by the use of whole-wheat pasta shells and low-fat cheeses, while gaining fiber and maintaining flavor with the addition of spinach and butternut squash. There's no need to precook the shells in this simple and delicious traditional Italian pasta meal.

Serves 6

2 cups cubed butternut squash

1 cup frozen spinach, thawed and squeezed dry

1 cup low-fat cottage cheese

1 cup part-skim ricotta cheese

½ cup grated Parmesan cheese

2 tablespoons Italian seasoning

Nonstick cooking spray

6 cups Rustic Marinara Sauce (page 16) or jarred sauce, divided

1 cup water

1 (12-ounce) package jumbo whole-wheat pasta shells

1. Place the butternut squash in a microwave-safe bowl and microwave on high for 4 to 5 minutes, or until soft. Transfer the squash to a large bowl and mash it with a fork. Add the spinach, cottage cheese, ricotta, Parmesan, and Italian seasoning and mix well. The mixture will be stiff.

2. Spray the inside of a 6-quart slow cooker with the cooking spray. Mix 2 cups of marinara sauce with the water in the bottom of the slow cooker. Fill each pasta shell with cheese-and-vegetable mixture and layer half of them in the bottom of the slow cooker, open-side up. Spoon another 2 cups of marinara sauce over the shells. Repeat with the remaining shells and the remaining 2 cups of marinara sauce.

3. Cover and cook on low for 6 to 8 hours.

4. Serve hot, with additional cheeses and fresh basil, if desired.

Per Serving (5 to 6 shells): Calories: 391; Total Fat: 10g; Saturated Fat: 4g; Trans Fat: 0g; Polyunsaturated Fat: 1g; Monounsaturated Fat: 1g; Cholesterol: 12mg; Sodium: 397mg; Carbohydrates: 54g; Fiber: 7g; Sugars: 7g; Protein: 22g

MAKE-AHEAD: To make these a freezer meal, assemble the shells into a glass dish including the top layer of sauce, then cover and freeze. When you are ready to cook the shells, allow them to thaw overnight, then place in your slow cooker following the steps above.

WHITE BEAN CABBAGE CASSEROLE

Prep time: 15 minutes / Cook time: 7 to 8 hours on low

This vegan version of stuffed cabbage replaces ground meat with creamy white beans in a casserole-like dish. Although it has all the flavor of traditional stuffed cabbage, this slow cooker version is much simpler to make.

Serves 6

2 (15-ounce) cans cannellini beans, drained and rinsed, or 1½ to 2 cups Savory Great Northern Beans (page 56)

1 small head of cabbage, cored and leaves sliced (about 5 to 6 cups total)

1 (14.5-ounce) can no-salt-added diced tomatoes

2 cups riced cauliflower

1 cup Savory Vegetable Broth (page 24) or low-sodium vegetable broth

1 onion, diced

4 garlic cloves, finely chopped

2 tablespoons extra-virgin olive oil

1 tablespoon Italian seasoning

1 teaspoon smoked paprika

Freshly ground black pepper

1. Combine all the ingredients to a 6-quart slow cooker. Cover and cook on low for 7 to 8 hours.

2. Serve hot.

Per Serving (1⅔ cups): Calories: 202; Total Fat: 5g; Saturated Fat: 1g; Trans Fat: 0g; Polyunsaturated Fat: 1g; Monounsaturated Fat: 3g; Cholesterol: 0mg; Sodium: 51mg; Carbohydrates: 30g; Fiber: 9g; Sugars: 7g; Protein: 10g

COOKING TIP: You can use frozen cauliflower rice or pulse raw cauliflower florets in your food processor until it resembles the texture of rice. Brown rice can also be used for a more traditional cabbage casserole. Use 1 cup of uncooked brown rice and 2 cups of vegetable broth or water to the casserole before cooking.

QUINOA AND BEAN-STUFFED PEPPERS

Prep time: 15 minutes / Cook time: 7 to 8 hours on low

These quinoa and bean-stuffed peppers can be made with basic pantry ingredients and minimal prep for a great meatless Monday dish. Quinoa adds a nutty flavor to the delicious filling of beans, onions, mushrooms, and more. If you don't like quinoa, just substitute brown rice instead. Top off this dish with a Creamy Queso Dip (page 21) for added flavor and nutrition.

Serves 6

6 large green, red, orange, or yellow bell peppers, or a combination

2 (15-ounce) cans black beans, drained and rinsed

1 cup quinoa, rinsed

1 cup chopped onion

1 cup chopped button mushrooms

½ cup chopped red bell pepper

1 cup Spicy Salsa (page 19)

1 tablespoon chopped fresh cilantro

1 teaspoon ground cumin

1 cup Creamy Queso Dip (page 21) or 1 cup shredded low-fat cheese, divided

Nonstick cooking spray

½ cup water

Freshly ground black pepper

1. Cut the tops off the peppers using a small knife and remove the stem and seeds. Reach inside and pull out any white bits of membrane that may remain. If any peppers do not stand up on their own, slice a very small amount off the bottom to create a flat bottom (you don't want the bottoms to have holes in them, so slice as little off as possible).

2. In a large bowl, combine the beans, quinoa, onion, mushrooms, chopped bell pepper, salsa, cilantro, cumin, and ½ cup of queso. Fill each pepper with the quinoa mixture.

3. Spray the inside of a 6-quart slow cooker with the cooking spray. Pour ½ cup of water into the bottom of the slow cooker. Place the peppers in the slow cooker so they are sitting in the water. Cover and cook on low for 7 to 8 hours.

4. In the last 30 minutes of cooking, remove the lid and pour the remaining ½ cup of queso sauce over the peppers and cover again until everything is heated through.

5. Serve hot.

Per Serving (1 stuffed pepper): Calories: 320; Total Fat: 4g; Saturated Fat: 2g; Trans Fat: 0g; Polyunsaturated Fat: 1g; Monounsaturated Fat: 1g; Cholesterol: 5mg; Sodium: 105mg; Carbohydrates: 56g; Fiber: 9g; Sugars: 5g; Protein: 15g

VARIATION TIP: For a more Southwestern dish, replace the mushrooms or some of the beans with corn. You could also add green chiles, if desired.

VEGAN RED BEANS AND RICE

Prep time: 10 minutes, plus overnight to soak / Cook time: 7 to 8 hours on low

Although this red beans and rice recipe doesn't have sausage, it has all of the flavors you would expect from a traditional Cajun-style dish. This vegan version uses a dash of paprika to mimic the characteristic smoky flavor of the sausage.

Serves 8

1 pound dried kidney beans, soaked overnight and drained

6 cups Savory Vegetable Broth (page 24) or low-sodium vegetable broth

1 (14.5-ounce) can no-salt-added fire-roasted tomatoes

1 onion, diced

1 bell pepper (any color), diced

4 garlic cloves, minced

1 teaspoon Creole seasoning (or to taste)

2 bay leaves

1 teaspoon dried thyme

1 teaspoon dried oregano

½ teaspoon smoked paprika

2 cups brown rice, cooked according to package directions

1. Put the beans, broth, tomatoes, onion, bell pepper, garlic, Creole seasoning, bay leaves, thyme, oregano, and paprika in a 6-quart slow cooker and stir to combine. Cover and cook on low for 7 to 8 hours.

2. Remove and discard the bay leaves. Serve hot over the brown rice.

Per Serving (2 cups): Calories: 380; Total Fat: 1g; Saturated Fat: 0g; Trans Fat: 0g; Polyunsaturated Fat: 0g; Monounsaturated Fat: 0g; Cholesterol: 0mg; Sodium: 196mg; Carbohydrates: 75g; Fiber: 12g; Sugars: 5g; Protein: 17g

VARIATION TIP: During the last 2 hours of cooking, add extra vegetables if you wish. Zucchini, eggplant, carrots, winter squash, and mushrooms are all great choices.

BUTTERNUT SQUASH MACARONI AND CHEESE

Prep time: 15 minutes / Cook time: 6 to 8 hours on low, plus 30 minutes on high

Macaroni and cheese is a classic comfort food loved by many. This version uses creamy butternut squash to add fiber, vitamins, and minerals while keeping calories and unhealthy fats in check. Whole-wheat macaroni adds energy-sustaining complex carbohydrates to a comfort food you can feel good about eating.

Serves 6

4 cups cubed butternut squash

3 cups Savory Vegetable Broth (page 24) or low-sodium vegetable broth

2 cup low-fat or fat-free milk, or unsweetened almond milk

1 medium onion, diced

4 garlic cloves, minced

1 teaspoon dried yellow mustard

½ teaspoon smoked paprika

3 cups whole-wheat elbow macaroni

1 cup low-fat shredded Cheddar cheese

1. Put the squash, broth, milk, onion, garlic, mustard, and paprika in a 6-quart slow cooker and stir well. Cover and cook on low for 6 to 8 hours.

2. Blend the sauce with an immersion blender (or in small batches in a regular blender) until smooth. Stir the pasta into the slow cooker and cook on high for 30 minutes, or until the pasta is al dente.

3. Stir in the cheese until melted. Serve hot.

Per Serving (1½ cups): Calories: 348; Total Fat: 6g; Saturated Fat: 2g; Trans Fat: 0g; Polyunsaturated Fat: 1g; Monounsaturated Fat: 1g; Cholesterol: 10mg; Sodium: 287mg; Carbohydrates: 60g; Fiber: 10g; Sugars: 7g; Protein: 14g

VARIATION TIP: You can also cook the pasta separately on the stove top and just pour the sauce over the cooked pasta to reduce the amount of finishing time for the recipe.

ALLERGY-FREE • VEGAN

THREE-BEAN CHILI

Prep time: 10 minutes / Cook time: 7 to 8 hours on low

Chili is one of those dishes that can vary: from super simple, to those with "secret ingredients," to ones that require an enormous shopping list. This mild family-friendly chili recipe is simple, yet delicious and you can prep it in minutes and then let the slow cooker do the work. There's no secret ingredient or two-hour shopping trip involved.

Serves 6

1 (15-ounce) can black beans, drained and rinsed

1 (15-ounce) can pinto beans, drained and rinsed

2 (15-ounce) cans kidney beans, drained and rinsed

2 (14.5-ounce) cans no-salt-added fire-roasted tomatoes

2 cups Savory Vegetable Broth (page 24) or low-sodium vegetable broth

1½ cups corn kernels

1 red bell pepper, chopped

1 green bell pepper, chopped

2 onions, chopped

4 garlic cloves, minced

½ cup Spicy Salsa (page 19)

1 tablespoon ground cumin

1 tablespoon chili powder (or more to taste)

1 teaspoon dried oregano

1. Combine all the ingredients in a 6-quart slow cooker. Cover and cook on low for 7 to 8 hours.

2. Serve hot with your favorite chili toppings.

Per Serving (2 cups): Calories: 317; Total Fat: 0g; Saturated Fat: 0g; Trans Fat: 0g; Polyunsaturated Fat: 0g; Monounsaturated Fat: 0g; Cholesterol: 0mg; Sodium: 380mg; Carbohydrates: 61g; Fiber: 15g; Sugars: 12g; Protein: 17g

COOKING TIP: You could also substitute 1 to 2 cans of beans with chili beans in their sauces. If you do this, wait to add the broth until the end of the cooking time, and adjust the amount of liquid depending on how thick or thin you like your chili.

ALLERGY-FREE • VEGAN

LENTIL BOLOGNESE

Prep time: 15 minutes / Cook time: 7 to 8 hours on low

This healthy and simple lentil Bolognese is full of fiber and plant-powered protein and makes a satisfying meal any night of the week. French lentilles du Puy give the sauce a meaty consistency while mushrooms lend an umami flavor. Vegan and allergy-free, this delicious and healthy dish full is of traditional Italian flavors.

Serves 8

1 pound lentilles du Puy, rinsed and picked through

4 cups Savory Vegetable Broth (page 24) or low-sodium vegetable broth

2 (28-ounce) cans crushed tomatoes

4 shallots, diced

2 medium carrots, diced

2 celery stalks, diced

1 cup sliced button mushrooms

6 garlic cloves, minced

2 bay leaves

2 tablespoons dried basil

1 tablespoon dried oregano

1 tablespoon extra-virgin olive oil

1 teaspoon dried marjoram

1 teaspoon crushed red pepper flakes

1. Combine all the ingredients in a 6-quart slow cooker. Cover and cook on low for 7 to 8 hours, until lentils and vegetables are tender and the sauce has thickened.

2. Serve hot over whole-wheat pasta, vegetable noodles, or your favorite grains.

Per Serving (2 cups): Calories: 300; Total Fat: 2g; Saturated Fat: 0g; Trans Fat: 0g; Polyunsaturated Fat: 1g; Monounsaturated Fat: 1g; Cholesterol: 0mg; Sodium: 384mg; Carbohydrates: 51g; Fiber: 21g; Sugars: 9g; Protein: 19g

COOKING TIP: French lentilles du Puy hold up best to slow cooking. However, the more common brown lentils are a perfectly delicious substitute.

VEGGIE FAJITAS

Prep time: 10 minutes / Cook time: 7 to 8 hours on low

This budget-friendly veggie fajita dish is sure to be a family hit. Black beans, peppers, onions, and tomatoes slow cook in traditional fajita seasonings so that when you get home you simply serve with flour tortillas and your favorite toppings. Bold flavors don't require a fat wallet!

Serves 6

1 (15-ounce) can black beans, drained and rinsed

1 (14.5-ounce) can fire-roasted tomatoes

4 medium red, orange, or yellow bell peppers or a mix, sliced

1 large onion, sliced

1 (4-ounce) can green chiles

4 garlic cloves, minced

1 tablespoon extra-virgin olive oil

1 tablespoon ground cumin

1 teaspoon dried oregano

Freshly ground black pepper

1. Combine all the ingredients in a 6-quart slow cooker. Cover and cook on low for 7 to 8 hours.

2. Serve hot.

Per Serving (¾ cup): Calories: 152; Total Fat: 3g; Saturated Fat: 0g; Trans Fat: 0g; Polyunsaturated Fat: 0g; Monounsaturated Fat: 2g; Cholesterol: 0mg; Sodium: 132mg; Carbohydrates: 26g; Fiber: 6g; Sugars: 6g; Protein: 7g

MAKE-AHEAD: You can prep and freeze part of this meal ahead of time by combining the sliced peppers, onions, garlic, beans, and spices and storing them in a freezer-safe bag. The night before you want to eat your fajitas, take the bag out of the freezer and thaw it in the refrigerator overnight. In the morning, simply add the veggie mix to the slow cooker along with the tomatoes, chiles, and oil.

VEGGIE LASAGNA

Prep time: 15 minutes / Cook time: 6½ to 7½ hours on low

This no-fuss lasagna recipe doesn't require precooking the noodles, which considerably cuts down on the amount of work involved. This recipe is easy to customize with your favorite vegetables and mix of cheeses. The use of homemade marinara sauce eliminates the sugar and salt found in jarred versions, making this a protein- and fiber-rich heart-healthy dish the whole family will enjoy.

Serves 6

Nonstick cooking spray

4 cups Rustic Marinara Sauce (page 16), divided

8 whole-wheat lasagna noodles

1½ cups part-skim ricotta cheese, divided

¾ cup green peas, thawed if frozen, divided

3 cups baby spinach, divided

3 cups sliced zucchini, divided

1 cup frozen butternut squash purée, thawed, divided

3 portobello mushroom caps, gills removed and thinly sliced, divided

½ cup shredded part-skim mozzarella cheese, divided

1. Lightly spray the inside of a 6-quart slow cooker with the cooking spray. Spread ½ cup of marinara sauce on the bottom of the slow cooker. Add a layer of noodles, trying not to overlap them. Break them into pieces, if necessary, to fully cover the bottom. Cover the noodles with ½ cup of ricotta cheese, ¼ cup of green peas, 1 cup of spinach, 1 cup of zucchini, ⅓ cup of squash purée, 1 sliced mushroom, and ¾ cup of marinara sauce. Repeat these layers twice more for three layers total. End with a final layer of noodles, the remaining ¼ cup of marinara sauce, and the mozzarella cheese.

2. Cover and cook on low for 6 to 7 hours. Then turn the slow cooker off and let the lasagna set for 30 minutes before serving to allow the noodles to firm up.

3. Serve hot.

Per Serving (1½ cups): Calories: 364; Total Fat: 11g; Saturated Fat: 5g; Trans Fat: 0g; Polyunsaturated Fat: 1g; Monounsaturated Fat: 2g; Cholesterol: 29mg; Sodium: 315mg; Carbohydrates: 48g; Fiber: 10g; Sugars: 10g; Protein: 20g

SUBSTITUTION TIP: You can make this dish gluten-free by using gluten-free lasagna noodles in place of wheat-based noodles. Find them at most supermarkets.

FRITTATA WITH SPINACH AND ROASTED PEPPERS

Prep time: 10 minutes / Cook time: 3 to 4 hours on low

Eggs are a high-quality, nutritious source of protein and are versatile enough to create filling breakfasts, lunches, and dinners. This recipe is virtually effortless. Eggs, rich-tasting roasted red peppers, cheese, and fiber-dense spinach are combined to create a filling frittata without the fuss.

Serves 6

Nonstick cooking spray

12 large eggs, well beaten

⅓ cup low-fat or fat-free milk, or plant-based milk

2 teaspoons extra-virgin olive oil

1 teaspoon dried thyme

4 cups packed chopped baby spinach, stemmed

1½ cups chopped Roasted Peppers (page 148)

½ cup chopped scallions

1 medium tomato, seeded and chopped

½ cup low-fat grated Cheddar cheese

1. Coat the inside of a 6-quart slow cooker with the cooking spray.

2. In a medium bowl, whisk together the eggs, milk, olive oil, and thyme.

3. Place the spinach, peppers, scallions, and tomato in the slow cooker. Pour the egg mixture over the vegetables. Sprinkle the cheese on top.

4. Cover and cook on low for 3 to 4 hours, until the frittata is well set and a knife inserted in the center comes out clean.

5. Serve hot, with a green salad and crusty bread.

Per Serving (1 cup): Calories: 212; Total Fat: 13g; Saturated Fat: 5g; Trans Fat: 0g; Polyunsaturated Fat: 2g; Monounsaturated Fat: 5g; Cholesterol: 379mg; Sodium: 251mg; Carbohydrates: 6g; Fiber: 2g; Sugars: 3g; Protein: 16g

COOKING TIP: This recipe freezes well for grab-and-go healthy breakfasts and lunches. Allow the frittata to cool, then cut it into equal-size square portions. Divide among freezer-safe resealable bags and freeze for up to 3 months.

CHICKPEA TIKKA MASALA

Prep time: 10 minutes / Cook time: 7 to 8 hours on low

A well-known Indian dish, tikka masala is delicious but unfortunately is high in calories and fat because of the heavy cream used in traditional recipes. This lightened-up, heart-healthy, vegan version uses light coconut milk and ramps up the fiber and nutrients by adding cauliflower and chickpeas.

Serves 6

1 (28-ounce) can no-salt-added fire-roasted tomatoes

3 (15-ounce) cans chickpeas, drained and rinsed

1 cup Savory Vegetable Broth (page 24), low-sodium vegetable broth, or water

1 cup green peas (thawed if frozen)

1 onion, diced

1 red bell pepper, diced

4 garlic cloves, minced

2 tablespoons tomato paste

2 tablespoons garam masala

1 tablespoon minced ginger

2 teaspoons extra-virgin olive oil

Freshly ground black pepper

4 cups cauliflower florets

1 (13.5-ounce) can light coconut milk

1. Put the tomatoes, chickpeas, broth, peas, onion, bell pepper, garlic, tomato paste, garam masala, ginger, olive oil, and black pepper in a 6-quart slow cooker and stir. Cover and cook on low for 7 to 8 hours.

2. Stir in the cauliflower and coconut milk with 30 minutes left of cooking time. Leave the slow cooker uncovered to finish cooking and thicken the sauce.

3. Serve hot over rice, if desired.

Per Serving (2 cups): Calories: 304; Total Fat: 5g; Saturated Fat: 3g; Trans Fat: 0g; Polyunsaturated Fat: 1g; Monounsaturated Fat: 1g; Cholesterol: 0mg; Sodium: 434mg; Carbohydrates: 48g; Fiber: 14g; Sugars: 9g; Protein: 16g

COOKING TIP: Garam masala typically contains a mix of black and white peppercorns, cloves, cinnamon, mace, black and green cardamom pods, bay leaf, cumin, and coriander.

CHICKPEA SLOPPY JOES

Prep time: 10 minutes / Cook time: 7 to 8 hours on low

This vegan sloppy Joe recipe has the same tangy great taste as traditional ground beef sloppy Joes, but it is made without unhealthy fats and added sugars. Lentils are used as the base with added chickpeas and veggies, which are covered in a homemade tangy sauce to create a dish full of flavor and heart-healthy nutrients.

Serves 6

4 cups Savory Vegetable
    Broth (page 24) or low-
    sodium vegetable broth

2 (15-ounce) cans chickpeas,
    drained and rinsed

1 cup brown lentils, rinsed
    and picked over

1 cup Rustic Marinara
    Sauce (page 16)

2 medium carrots, diced

1 medium onion, diced

1 bell pepper (any color), diced

4 garlic cloves, minced

4 tablespoons tomato paste

1 tablespoon molasses

1 tablespoon apple cider vinegar

½ tablespoon dried mustard
    (or more to taste)

Freshly ground black pepper

1. Combine all the ingredients to a 6-quart slow cooker. Cover and cook on low for 7 to 8 hours until the lentils are tender and the sauce has thickened.

2. In the last 30 minutes of cooking, open the slow cooker and mash one-quarter to one-third of the filling with a potato masher. Stir, cover, and cook for the remaining 30 minutes.

3. Serve hot on toasted whole-wheat buns with your favorite toppings or in lettuce leaves, if desired.

Per Serving (1½ cups): Calories: 262; Total Fat: 0g; Saturated Fat: 0g; Trans Fat: 0g; Polyunsaturated Fat: 0g; Monounsaturated Fat: 0g; Cholesterol: 0mg; Sodium: 215mg; Carbohydrates: 49g; Fiber: 15g; Sugars: 10g; Protein: 14g

NUTRITIONAL HIGHLIGHT: Molasses is unlike refined sugar in that it has nutritional benefits. Blackstrap molasses contains iron, calcium, magnesium, vitamin B6, and selenium. It is also digested more slowly than sugar, making it a diabetes-friendly sweetener.

MUSHROOM STROGANOFF

Prep time: 15 minutes / Cook time: 7½ hours on low

You won't miss the beef in this vegetarian slow cooker recipe for mushroom stroganoff. The long cooking time allows the mushrooms to create a decadent sauce that is lightened up with the use of light sour cream. You can serve this delicious, comforting meal over rice or the more traditional egg noodles.

Serves 6

1 tablespoon extra-virgin olive oil

2 pounds mushrooms, sliced (see Cooking Tip)

1 large onion, diced

3 garlic cloves, minced

3 cups Savory Vegetable Broth (page 24) or low-sodium vegetable broth, divided

4 tablespoons Homemade Ketchup (page 20)

1 teaspoon smoked paprika

½ teaspoon freshly ground black pepper

¾ cup low-fat sour cream

1 tablespoon cornstarch

4 cups baby spinach

1. Add the olive oil, mushrooms, onion, and garlic to a 6-quart slow cooker.

2. In a large bowl, mix together 2½ cups of broth, the ketchup, paprika, and black pepper. Pour this over the mushrooms. Cover and cook on low for 7½ hours.

3. With 30 minutes of cooking time left, in a small bowl, combine the sour cream, cornstarch, and remaining ½ cup of broth. Stir this into the slow cooker along with the spinach. Cover and cook on low for 30 minutes until the sauce has thickened and spinach has wilted.

4. Serve hot over rice or noodles.

Per Serving (1 cup): Calories: 134; Total Fat: 5g; Saturated Fat: 2g; Trans Fat: 0g; Polyunsaturated Fat: 1g; Monounsaturated Fat: 2g; Cholesterol: 8mg; Sodium: 136mg; Carbohydrates: 16g; Fiber: 3g; Sugars: 10g; Protein: 7g

COOKING TIP: You can use any combination of mushrooms you like. Aim for a variety such as baby Portabellos, cremini, white button, oyster, shiitake, or even some dried porcinis.

WILD RICE AND EGG CASSEROLE

Prep time: 10 minutes / Cook time: 5 to 6 hours on low

Healthy "fried rice"—who knew!? This easy, healthy, and nutritious vegetarian main dish combines the contrasting textures of chewy wild rice and soft and meaty mushrooms and eggs. Feel free to swap out the seasonings for your favorites.

Serves 6

2 cups wild rice blend

1 tablespoon extra-virgin olive oil

4 cups Savory Vegetable Broth (page 24) or low-sodium vegetable broth

4 scallions, white and green parts, chopped

1 cup sliced button mushrooms

1 cup quartered Brussels sprouts

2 garlic cloves, minced

2 teaspoons dried sage

Freshly ground black pepper

2 large eggs, whisked

2 large egg whites, whisked

1. Put the rice and oil in a 6-quart slow cooker and stir to coat the rice grains well. Add the broth, scallions, mushrooms, Brussels sprouts, garlic, sage, and black pepper. Pour in the eggs and egg whites and stir to combine.

2. Cover and cook on low for 5 to 6 hours, until the rice and vegetables are tender and the eggs are set.

3. Serve hot.

Per Serving (1⅓ cups): Calories: 253; Total Fat: 3g; Saturated Fat: 1g; Trans Fat: 0g; Polyunsaturated Fat: 1g; Monounsaturated Fat: 1g; Cholesterol: 62mg; Sodium: 141mg; Carbohydrates: 49g; Fiber: 4g; Sugars: 3g; Protein: 12g

COOKING TIP: For a more traditional fried rice flavor, replace the sage with Chinese five-spice powder, add minced fresh ginger, and serve with low-sodium soy sauce.

SPICY BEAN AND RICE–STUFFED PEPPERS

Prep time: 15 minutes / Cook time: 7 to 8 hours on low

No stove top prep with these stuffed peppers! Simply mix, stuff, and walk away! The Mexican spin on stuffed peppers has never been better for your heart.

Serves 6

1 (15-ounce) can no-salt-added black beans, drained and rinsed

1 (15-ounce) can no-salt-added pinto beans, drained and rinsed

1 (4-ounce) can diced green chiles

1¼ cups Spicy Salsa (page 19) or store-bought salsa

1 cup frozen corn

1 cup quick-cooking (Minute) brown rice

1 cup 2% shredded Cheddar cheese, divided

2 teaspoons ground cumin

2 teaspoons chili powder

6 bell peppers (any color), tops cut off, seeded, membrane removed

1 cup water

1. In a large bowl, mix together the black beans, pinto beans, chiles, salsa, corn, rice, ¾ cup of cheese, cumin, and chili powder. Fill each bell pepper with the mixture and stand each pepper in a 6-quart slow cooker top-side up. Pour the water in the space between the peppers, being careful not to pour it over the peppers or filling.

2. Cover and cook on low for 7 to 8 hours.

3. Sprinkle each pepper with the remaining ¼ cup of cheese. Cover the slow cooker and cook an additional 3 to 4 minutes, or until cheese is melted.

4. Serve hot.

Per Serving (1 stuffed pepper): Calories: 294; Total Fat: 5g; Saturated Fat: 3g; Trans Fat: 0g; Polyunsaturated Fat: 1g; Monounsaturated Fat: 1g; Cholesterol: 13mg; Sodium: 396mg; Carbohydrates: 52g; Fiber: 10g; Sugars: 7g; Protein: 16g

SUBSTITUTION TIP: If you want additional spice, add chipotle peppers in adobo, which can be found in small cans in the ethnic food aisle of most supermarkets. These peppers pack big punch!

VEGETABLE CURRY

Prep time: 15 minutes / Cook time: 7 to 8 hours on low

This creamy and delicious Indian-influenced vegetable curry is packed with plant protein from chickpeas and green peas and full of flavor from the mix of warm spices. Feel free to add additional vegetables or swap out the chickpeas for your favorite type of bean. The sky's the limit.

Serves 6 to 8

1 (28-ounce) can no-salt-added diced tomatoes

1 (15-ounce) can chickpeas, drained and rinsed

1 (14-ounce) can light coconut milk

4 cups cauliflower florets

2 cups Savory Vegetable Broth (page 24) or low-sodium vegetable broth

1 cup sliced carrots

2 red bell peppers, diced

1 medium sweet potato, peeled and diced

1 large onion, diced

2 tablespoons grated fresh ginger

1 tablespoon curry powder

1 tablespoon turmeric

4 garlic cloves, minced

Freshly ground black pepper

Pinch cayenne pepper (optional)

1½ cups frozen peas

1. Put the tomatoes, chickpeas, coconut milk, cauliflower, broth, carrots, bell peppers, sweet potato, onion, ginger, curry powder, turmeric, garlic, pepper, and cayenne pepper (if using) in a 6-quart slow cooker and stir to combine. Cover and cook on low for 7 to 8 hours, until the vegetables are tender.

2. Before serving, stir in the peas and let stand until warmed through.

3. Serve over brown rice or grain of choice.

Per Serving (1¾ cups): Calories: 277; Total Fat: 8g; Saturated Fat: 4g; Trans Fat: 0g; Polyunsaturated Fat: 1g; Monounsaturated Fat: 0g; Cholesterol: 0mg; Sodium: 178mg; Carbohydrates: 44g; Fiber: 11g; Sugars: 14g; Protein: 10g

NUTRITIONAL HIGHLIGHT: Curry powder is made from a collection of spices usually including cumin, turmeric, cinnamon, cloves, and others. The substance called curcumin in turmeric has been studied for its inflammation-reducing properties.

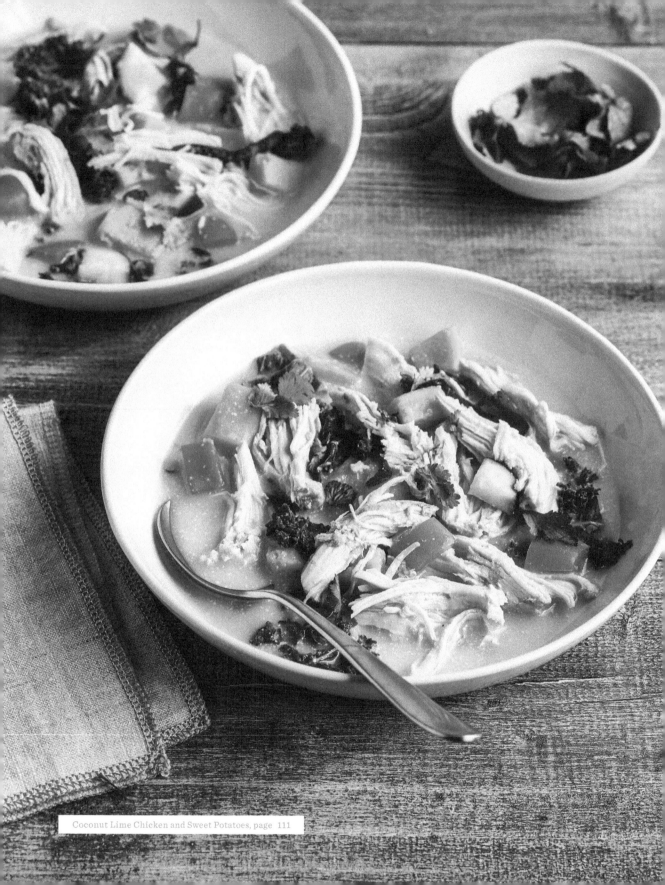

Coconut Lime Chicken and Sweet Potatoes, page 111

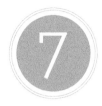

Poultry Mains

SHREDDED CHICKEN SLOPPY JOES

Prep time: 15 minutes / Cook time: 6 to 7 hours on low

These spicy, shredded chicken sloppy Joes are made with a delicious and unique twist—finely chopped dates add a touch of sweetness to balance the spice without the use of added sugars. Enjoy on a whole-grain bun, or keep this dish light and serve in a lettuce wrap or over a bed of greens.

Serves 8

2 pounds boneless, skinless chicken breasts

1 (14-ounce) can tomato sauce

1 cup finely shredded carrots

4 dates, pitted and finely chopped

¼ cup tomato paste

1 jalapeño pepper, seeded and diced

4 garlic cloves, minced

3 tablespoons yellow mustard

2 tablespoons apple cider vinegar

1 teaspoon chili powder

1 teaspoon onion powder

Freshly ground black pepper

1. Combine all the ingredients in a 6-quart slow cooker. Cover and cook on low for 6 to 7 hours.

2. Remove the chicken from the slow cooker and shred it with two forks. Return the chicken to the slow cooker, stir to mix, and continue cooking until ready to serve.

3. Serve hot.

Per Serving (1 cup): Calories: 182; Total Fat: 4g; Saturated Fat: 1g; Trans Fat: 0g; Polyunsaturated Fat: 1g; Monounsaturated Fat: 2g; Cholesterol: 65mg; Sodium: 484mg; Carbohydrates: 9g; Fiber: 2g; Sugars: 6g; Protein: 28g

NUTRITIONAL HIGHLIGHT: Dates are an incredibly versatile and nutritious food. A good source of fiber, vitamins, and minerals, their sweetness can take the place of refined sugars in many recipes. Just be certain to chop them finely.

BALSAMIC CHICKEN AND VEGETABLES

Prep time: 5 minutes / Cook time: 7 to 8 hours on low

This balsamic chicken and vegetables is simple to prep and rich in satiating protein, fiber, and health-promoting vitamins and minerals. Balsamic vinegar contains antioxidants that can protect the body from chronic diseases like heart disease. Baby red potatoes, carrots, and tomatoes make this a filling and satisfying one-pot meal.

Serves 6

1 tablespoon extra-virgin olive oil

4 garlic cloves, minced

1 pound baby red potatoes, halved

2 cups sliced carrots

6 boneless, skinless chicken breasts (about 1½ pounds)

½ cup balsamic vinegar

½ cup Chicken Stock (page 25) or low-sodium chicken broth

¼ cup honey

1 teaspoon dried thyme

1 teaspoon dried rosemary

½ teaspoon dried oregano

1 (14.5-ounce) can no-salt-added diced tomatoes, slightly drained

1. Spread the oil and garlic in the bottom of a 6-quart slow cooker. Layer in the potatoes, followed by the carrots, then place the chicken on top.

2. In a small bowl, whisk together the vinegar, stock, honey, thyme, rosemary, and oregano. Pour the mixture over the chicken. Top with the tomatoes.

3. Cover and cook on low for 7 to 8 hours, until the chicken is cooked through and the vegetables are tender.

4. Serve with your favorite green vegetables.

Per Serving (1 chicken breast plus 1 cup vegetables): Calories: 284; Total Fat: 5g; Saturated Fat: 1g; Trans Fat: 0g; Polyunsaturated Fat: 1g; Monounsaturated Fat: 2g; Cholesterol: 70mg; Sodium: 534mg; Carbohydrates: 35g; Fiber: 3g; Sugars: 15g; Protein: 25g

VARIATION TIP: If you will be near your slow cooker during the last 30 minutes, add 1 pound of chopped green beans, cover and cook until tender.

JAMAICAN JERK CHICKEN AND BLACK BEANS

Prep time: 5 minutes / Cook time: 6 to 8 hours on low

This jerk chicken recipe serves up nicely with your favorite sautéed vegetables and some coconut rice or baked sweet potatoes. Chicken thighs are used in this recipe but chicken breasts would work just as well. The mix of spices, with just the right amount of heat, makes this a fragrant and flavorful dish.

Serves 6

3 to 4 pounds boneless, skinless chicken thighs (about 2 thighs per person)

1 (15-ounce) can black beans, drained and rinsed

1 onion, sliced

1 bell pepper (any color), sliced

½ cup water

¼ cup honey

Juice of 3 limes

4 garlic cloves, minced

1 tablespoon extra-virgin olive oil

1 teaspoon freshly ground black pepper

1 teaspoon allspice

1 teaspoon dried thyme

½ teaspoon ground cinnamon

½ teaspoon chili powder

Pinch cayenne pepper

1. Place the chicken, beans, onion, and bell pepper in a 6-quart slow cooker.

2. In a small bowl, mix together the water, honey, lime juice, garlic, oil, black pepper, allspice, thyme, cinnamon, chili powder, and cayenne pepper. Pour this over the chicken, beans, and vegetables. Stir to coat the chicken and vegetables.

3. Cover and cook on low for 6 to 8 hours, until the chicken is cooked through.

Per Serving (2 thighs plus ⅓ cup bean-and-vegetable mixture): Calories: 438; Total Fat: 16g; Saturated Fat: 4g; Trans Fat: 0g; Polyunsaturated Fat: 1g; Monounsaturated Fat: 2g; Cholesterol: 130mg; Sodium: 182mg; Carbohydrates: 25g; Fiber: 3g; Sugars: 14g; Protein: 46g

COOKING TIP: You can use store-bought jerk seasoning in place of the spices used in this recipe, but most are fairly high in sodium. You can save money by making your own mix, which you can customize to your preferences. Most blends include onion powder, garlic, thyme, allspice, cinnamon, chili powder, cayenne pepper, some type of sweetener, and often nutmeg and paprika.

INDIAN BUTTER CHICKEN

Prep time: 15 minutes / Cook time: 6 to 8 hours on low

Not every version of butter chicken uses butter: This dish gets its name because the chicken becomes soft as butter when slow cooked in an Indian-spiced sauce. Light coconut milk gives this heart-healthy version its creamy richness, and the delicious flavors and simple prep make this a perfect dinner for busy weeknights.

Serves 6

2 pounds boneless, skinless
    chicken breasts, cut
    into 2-inch pieces

1 (14.5-ounce) can light
    coconut milk

1 (6-ounce) can tomato paste

1 onion, diced

1 red bell pepper, diced

4 garlic cloves, minced

2 tablespoons freshly
    squeezed lemon juice

1 tablespoon grated fresh ginger

2 teaspoons curry powder

2 teaspoons garam masala

1 cup nonfat plain
    yogurt, divided

1. Combine the chicken, coconut milk, tomato paste, onion, bell pepper, garlic, lemon juice, ginger, curry powder, and garam masala juice in a 6-quart slow cooker. Cover and cook on low for 6 to 8 hours, until the chicken is cooked through and the vegetables are tender.

2. Fifteen minutes before serving, stir in ½ cup of yogurt.

3. Serve hot with a dollop of the remaining ½ cup of yogurt on each serving. If desired, serve over basmati or jasmine rice with a garnish of fresh cilantro.

Per Serving (1¼ cups): Calories: 288; Total Fat: 9g; Saturated Fat: 5g; Trans Fat: 0g; Polyunsaturated Fat: 1g; Monounsaturated Fat: 3g; Cholesterol: 88mg; Sodium: 359mg; Carbohydrates: 13g; Fiber: 2g; Sugars: 7g; Protein: 40g

COOKING TIP: For a finished dish that is lower in carbohydrates and calories, serve over riced cauliflower instead of regular rice. You can find riced cauliflower in the produce and freezer sections of most supermarkets, or make your own with a few pulses in a food processor.

SALSA VERDE CHICKEN

Prep time: 10 minutes / Cook time: 5 to 6 hours on low

This recipe for salsa verde chicken couldn't be easier. With just a handful of pantry ingredients and 10 minutes of prep, you can have a delicious dinner ready to serve in just hours while you go about your day. It's an ideal weekend meal. Serve this delicious chicken over lettuce or rice, in tacos, or as a filling for enchiladas.

Serves 6

Nonstick cooking spray

2 pounds boneless, skinless chicken breasts

2 cups salsa verde

1 (14.5-ounce) can no-salt-added fire-roasted tomatoes

1 (4-ounce) can green chiles

1 bell pepper (any color), chopped

2 teaspoons ground cumin

1 teaspoon dried oregano

Freshly ground black pepper

Optional toppings: chopped fresh cilantro, avocado slices, lime wedges, lettuce leaves

1. Spray the inside of a 6-quart slow cooker with the cooking spray. Place the chicken in the bottom of the slow cooker. Add the salsa verde, tomatoes, chiles, bell pepper, cumin, oregano, and black pepper, and stir to combine. Cover and cook on low for 5 to 6 hours.

2. Remove the chicken and shred it using two forks. Stir the shredded chicken back into the slow cooker and taste to adjust seasonings.

3. Serve hot, with toppings such as chopped fresh cilantro, avocado slices, or lime wedges, if desired.

Per Serving (1⅔ cups): Calories: 257; Total Fat: 5g; Saturated Fat: 2g; Trans Fat: 0g; Polyunsaturated Fat: 1g; Monounsaturated Fat: 2g; Cholesterol: 87mg; Sodium: 646mg; Carbohydrates: 14g; Fiber: 4g; Sugars: 3g; Protein: 34g

COOKING TIP: You can also use a hand mixer or stand mixer to shred the chicken.

KUNG PAO CHICKEN

Prep time: 15 minutes / Cook time: 6 to 7 hours on low

Picking up takeout on the way home from work after a long day seems tempting, but it's really not very time-consuming to prep your own much healthier version in the morning before you head to work. Full of colorful veggies and lean chicken breast, this recipe uses a lighter sauce than typical takeout versions to keep unhealthy fats and sodium in check.

Serves 6

Nonstick cooking spray
2 pounds boneless, skinless chicken breast, cut into 1-inch pieces
1 (8-ounce) can water chestnuts, drained
2 celery stalks, chopped
1 red bell pepper chopped
1 green bell pepper chopped
4 medium carrots, sliced
½ cup plus 2 tablespoons water, divided
¼ cup low-sodium soy sauce
¼ cup balsamic vinegar
4 tablespoons sriracha sauce (or to taste)
4 garlic cloves, minced
2 tablespoons honey (or to taste)
1 tablespoon freshly grated ginger
1 tablespoon sesame oil
2 tablespoons cornstarch
2 cups snow peas

1. Spray the inside of a slow cooker with the cooking spray. Add the chicken, water chestnuts, celery, bell peppers, and carrots.

2. In a small bowl, whisk together ½ cup water, the soy sauce, balsamic vinegar, sriracha, garlic, honey, ginger, and sesame oil. Pour this over the chicken and vegetables. Cover and cook on low for 5 to 6 hours.

3. About 20 minutes before serving, whisk together the corn-starch and remaining 2 tablespoons of water until the cornstarch is dissolved. Stir this into the slow cooker along with the snow peas and continue cooking until sauce has thickened, 15 to 20 minutes depending on how hot your slow cooker gets.

4. Serve hot over rice or vegetables noodles garnished with chopped nuts and chopped scallions, if desired.

Per Serving (1¾ cups): Calories: 312; Total Fat: 8g; Saturated Fat: 3g; Trans Fat: 0g; Polyunsaturated Fat: 1g; Monounsaturated Fat: 3g; Cholesterol: 87mg; Sodium: 587mg; Carbohydrates: 24g; Fiber: 4g; Sugars: 13g; Protein: 36g

COOKING TIP: If you prefer your peppers on the crunchy side, add them when you add the snow peas and cornstarch thickener. Likewise if you like your chicken crispier, sauté in a saucepan with oil before adding it to the slow cooker. If you like your chicken saucier, you can double the sauce ingredients.

CHICKEN PROVENÇAL WITH WHITE BEANS

Prep time: 15 minutes / Cook time: 6 to 7 hours on low

The word *Provençal* refers to the people and region of Provence in southern France. When referring to food, the term means "cooked in a sauce consisting of garlic, onions, mushrooms, tomatoes, olive oil, and herbs," although there is no single standard sauce. This Provençal version makes a slight change to the spices, using tarragon and oregano, but feel free to use thyme, basil, and/or parsley depending on your taste preferences.

Serves 6

2 pounds boneless, skinless chicken breasts

1 (28-ounce) can no-salt-added diced tomatoes

2 cups Chicken Stock (page 25) or low-sodium chicken stock

1 (15-ounce) can cannellini beans, drained and rinsed

1 cup white wine

2 onions, finely chopped

8 garlic cloves, minced

4 tablespoons tomato paste

2 tablespoons extra-virgin olive oil

2 teaspoons dried tarragon

2 teaspoons dried oregano

Freshly ground black pepper

Zest of 1 lemon

Juice of 1 lemon

½ cup Niçoise or Kalamata olives

½ cup fresh parsley, minced

1. Put the chicken, tomatoes, stock, beans, wine, onions, garlic, tomato paste, olive oil, tarragon, oregano, and black pepper in a 6-quart slow cooker. Cover and cook on low for 6 to 7 hours, until chicken is cooked through.

2. Garnish the chicken and sauce with the lemon zest and juice, olives, and fresh parsley. Serve over rice, if desired.

Per Serving (2 cups): Calories: 405; Total Fat: 13g; Saturated Fat: 3g; Trans Fat: 0g; Polyunsaturated Fat: 2g; Monounsaturated Fat: 6g; Cholesterol: 87mg; Sodium: 387mg; Carbohydrates: 27g; Fiber: 6g; Sugars: 10g; Protein: 40g

COOKING TIP: Sometimes an extra step can make a recipe even more delicious. If you have time, create the sauce by first heating a medium sauté pan over medium-high heat. Heat the oil and add the onion, garlic, and tomato paste, and cook until the onions are soft, 3 to 4 minutes. Add the wine and cook until it is reduced by about half, 4 to 5 minutes. Add this to the slow cooker with the other ingredients and continue with the recipe. You can also make this sauce ahead of time and add it when you are ready to cook the meal.

COCONUT LIME CHICKEN AND SWEET POTATOES

Prep time: 10 minutes / Cook time: 6 to 8 hours on low

This creamy and delicious dish couldn't be easier. The few minutes of prep time make it all worthwhile. Slow cooking the chicken in the creamy coconut cilantro sauce allows it to really absorb the flavors, making it melt-in-your-mouth delicious. This recipe includes sweet potatoes but you can swap them out for your other favorites, such as winter squash, carrots, or creamy pumpkin.

Serves 6

1 cup water

4 garlic cloves, minced

1 tablespoon minced fresh ginger

Juice of 2 limes

1 teaspoon turmeric

1 teaspoon ground cumin

1 teaspoon curry powder

1 teaspoon ground coriander

Freshly ground black pepper

3 pounds boneless, skinless chicken breasts

4 cups sweet potato cubes

1 red bell pepper, chopped

1 cup chopped fresh cilantro

1 (15-ounce) can light coconut milk

1. Pour the water, garlic, ginger, and lime juice into the slow cooker and stir.

2. In a small bowl, mix together the turmeric, cumin, curry, coriander, and black pepper. Season the chicken on all sides with this spice mix, and add the chicken and any remaining spice mix to the slow cooker. Top the chicken with the sweet potatoes, bell pepper, and cilantro and stir to combine. Cover and cook on low for 6 to 8 hours, until chicken is cooked through and the vegetables are tender. Add the coconut milk to the slow cooker and stir to combine.

3. Serve hot.

Per Serving (2 cups): Calories: 419; Total Fat: 10g; Saturated Fat: 4g; Trans Fat: 0g; Polyunsaturated Fat: 1g; Monounsaturated Fat: 1g; Cholesterol: 130mg; Sodium: 212mg; Carbohydrates: 26g; Fiber: 4g; Sugars: 5g; Protein: 55g

VARIATION TIP: If you want to add quick-cooking vegetables to this dish such as zucchini, broccoli, cauliflower, spinach, or kale, add them in the last 30 minutes of cooking.

BUFFALO-SEASONED CHICKEN WRAP

Prep time: 10 minutes / Cook time: 7 to 8 hours on low

This light version of Buffalo chicken uses a simple seasoning mix of chicken broth and hot sauce instead of high-calorie, high-sodium ranch dressing. Complete the meal by wrapping the chicken in lettuce leaves.

Serves 6

For the chicken
Nonstick cooking spray

2 pounds boneless, skinless chicken breasts

2 medium celery stalks, chopped

1 medium onion, chopped

2 garlic cloves, minced

2 cups Chicken Stock (page 25) low-sodium chicken broth

½ cup cayenne hot sauce

2 tablespoons honey

For the blue-cheese sauce
¼ cup plain nonfat Greek yogurt

¼ cup blue cheese crumbles

¼ cup low-fat or fat-free milk, or plant-based milk (or more as needed)

1 tablespoon freshly squeezed lemon juice

Cayenne hot sauce to taste

To serve
8 to 16 large lettuce leaves, such as Bibb or romaine

2 cups shredded carrots

To make the chicken
1. Spray the inside of a 6-quart slow cooker with cooking spray. Place the chicken in the slow cooker and top it with the celery, onion, and garlic.

2. In a medium bowl, whisk together the stock, hot sauce, and honey. Pour this over the chicken. Cover and cook on low for 6 to 8 hours.

3. Remove the chicken and shred it using two forks. Stir the shredded chicken back into the Buffalo sauce and let it soak up the flavors for 5 to 10 minutes.

To make the blue-cheese sauce
Whisk together the yogurt, blue cheese, milk, lemon juice, and hot sauce.

To serve
To serve, wrap the chicken, shredded carrots, and blue-cheese sauce in 8 large (or 16 small) lettuce leaves. Add additional hot sauce, if desired.

Per Serving (1 large wrap or 2 wraps): Calories: 273; Total Fat: 7g; Saturated Fat: 3g; Trans Fat: 0g; Polyunsaturated Fat: 1g; Monounsaturated Fat: 3g; Cholesterol: 92mg; Sodium: 211mg; Carbohydrates: 15g; Fiber: 2g; Sugars: 10g; Protein: 37g

VARIATION TIP: If you like a thicker buffalo sauce, whisk together ¼ cup of cold water and 2 tablespoons of cornstarch, stir this into the slow cooker with the shredded chicken, and allow the sauce to thicken.

SESAME HONEY CHICKEN

Prep time: 10 minutes / Cook time: 5 to 6 hours on low

This sesame honey chicken has just the right balance of sweet and savory flavors. A simple yet flavorful sauce can be made in minutes using pantry staples. This sauce coats and tenderizes the chicken during the slow-cooking process. Serve this nutritious dish, complete with fiber-rich veggies, over brown rice or your favorite whole grains.

Serves 6

Nonstick cooking spray

2 pounds boneless, skinless chicken breasts, cut into 1-inch pieces

2 cups frozen, shelled edamame

4 medium carrots, sliced

1 medium onion, chopped

½ cup cold water

2 tablespoons cornstarch

½ cup Chicken Stock (page 25) or low-sodium chicken broth

1 tablespoon sesame oil or extra-virgin olive oil

4 garlic cloves, minced

¼ cup low-sodium soy sauce

¼ cup honey

¼ cup tomato paste

¼ cup rice wine vinegar

3 cups broccoli florets

4 tablespoons sesame seeds, for garnish

1. Spray a 6-quart slow cooker with the cooking spray. Add the chicken, edamame, carrots, and onion.

2. In a small bowl, whisk together cold water and cornstarch. Add the stock, sesame oil, garlic, soy sauce, honey, tomato paste, and vinegar and whisk to combine. Pour the sauce over chicken.

3. Cover and cook on low for 5 to 6 hours. In the last 30 minutes of cooking, stir in the broccoli and continue cooking until the vegetables are tender and the chicken is cooked through.

4. Serve hot, garnished with the sesame seeds. Serve over brown rice, if desired.

Per Serving (2 cups): Calories: 419; Total Fat: 13g; Saturated Fat: 3g; Trans Fat: 0g; Polyunsaturated Fat: 3g; Monounsaturated Fat: 5g; Cholesterol: 87mg; Sodium: 574mg; Carbohydrates: 33g; Fiber: 7g; Sugars: 18g; Protein: 43g

SUBSTITUTION TIP: You can easily make this recipe gluten-free by replacing the soy sauce with tamari. Cornstarch is naturally gluten-free.

ROSEMARY LEMON CHICKEN WITH VEGETABLES

Prep time: 10 minutes / Cook time: 7 to 8 hours on low

This healthy and delicious rosemary chicken and vegetable recipe is a snap to make and requires next to no prep. The chicken stays moist and tender and soaks up the flavors from the lemon and rosemary and the potatoes cook up perfectly. Simply add a green vegetable and side salad and you have a lovely, heart-healthy, satisfying meal.

Serves 6

1 pound baby potatoes, halved

6 medium carrots,
    peeled and sliced

2 medium onions, sliced

Freshly ground black pepper

3 teaspoons dried
    rosemary, divided

2 pounds boneless, skinless
    chicken breasts

Juice of 2 lemons (about ½ cup)

1 cup Chicken Stock (page 25)
    or low-sodium chicken broth

4 fresh rosemary sprigs

4 garlic cloves, minced

1. Place the potatoes, carrots, and onions in the bottom of the slow cooker. Sprinkle them with black pepper and 1½ teaspoons of dried rosemary. Place the chicken on top of the vegetables.

2. Pour the lemon juice and stock over the chicken and vegetables. Place the fresh rosemary and garlic on top of the chicken. Cover and cook on low for 7 to 8 hours, until the chicken is cooked through and vegetables are tender.

3. Remove and discard the rosemary sprigs. Serve hot.

Per Serving (1¾ cups): Calories: 288; Total Fat: 5g; Saturated Fat: 2g; Trans Fat: 0g; Polyunsaturated Fat: 1g; Monounsaturated Fat: 3g; Cholesterol: 87mg; Sodium: 108mg; Carbohydrates: 23g; Fiber: 4g; Sugars: 6g; Protein: 36g

COOKING TIP: Another way to save a bit of time is to keep containers of chopped onions and garlic on hand. You can find prechopped vegetables and jars of minced garlic in the produce section of the grocery store. Or chop your own and store in air-tight containers in your refrigerator.

CHICKEN CACCIATORE

Prep time: 10 minutes / Cook time: 7 to 8 hours on low

Cacciatore is Italian for "hunter," and it refers to food prepared hunter-style with mushrooms and onions. Easy to prep and full of healthy, satisfying ingredients, this recipe is a classic and continues to be a family hit.

Serves 6

4 portobello mushrooms, stemmed, thinly sliced

1 cup sliced button mushrooms

1 (28-ounce) can no-salt-added diced tomatoes

1 (6-ounce) can tomato paste

2 bell peppers (any color), thinly sliced

1 onion, diced

4 garlic cloves, minced

2 teaspoons dried basil

2 teaspoons dried oregano

Freshly ground black pepper

2 pounds boneless, skinless chicken breasts or thighs

1. Put the mushrooms, tomatoes, tomato paste, bell peppers, onion, garlic, basil, oregano, and black pepper in a 6-quart slow cooker. Stir to mix well. Add the chicken and mix again. Cover and cook on low for 7 to 8 hours, until the chicken is cooked through and the vegetables are tender.

2. Serve hot, over couscous, quinoa, mashed potatoes, riced cauliflower, or whole-wheat pasta, if desired.

Per Serving (1¾ cups): Calories: 277; Total Fat: 3g; Saturated Fat: 1g; Trans Fat: 0g; Polyunsaturated Fat: 1g; Monounsaturated Fat: 1g; Cholesterol: 87mg; Sodium: 108mg; Carbohydrates: 26g; Fiber: 4g; Sugars: 5g; Protein: 38g

COOKING TIP: You can substitute 28 ounces of seasoned spaghetti sauce or Rustic Marinara Sauce (page 16) for the diced tomatoes and tomato paste. Depending on what herbs are in the sauce, you may not need to add the dried spices, or you may have to reduce their amounts.

CHICKEN SPAGHETTI WITH PEPPERS AND ONIONS

Prep time: 10 minutes / Cook time: 4 hours on high or 7 to 8 hours on low

Ahh, spaghetti. Just the word makes many people perk up with anticipation. This healthy twist on spaghetti and meat sauce uses lean chicken breast and sneaks in bell peppers and onions to make the meal filling, rich in vitamins, and high in fiber.

Serves 6

Nonstick cooking spray

1½ pounds boneless, skinless chicken breasts (about 6 breasts)

1 green bell pepper, sliced

1 onion, halved and sliced

1 (28-ounce) can crushed tomatoes

1 (14-ounce) can no-salt-added diced tomatoes

4 garlic cloves, minced

1 tablespoon balsamic vinegar

1 teaspoon dried oregano

1 teaspoon Italian seasoning

12 ounces whole-wheat spaghetti

1. Spray a 6-quart slow cooker with the cooking spray. Place the chicken breasts in the bottom and top them with the sliced bell pepper and onion.

2. In a large bowl, mix together the crushed tomatoes, diced tomatoes, garlic, vinegar, oregano, and Italian seasoning. Pour this over the chicken and vegetables.

3. Cover and cook on high for 4 hours or on low for 7 to 8 hours.

4. Before serving, cook the pasta according to the package directions, omitting the salt and any fat. Serve the chicken and sauce over the cooked pasta.

Per Serving (1 cup pasta with ¾ cup sauce): Calories: 398; Total Fat: 6g; Saturated Fat: 2g; Trans Fat: 0g; Polyunsaturated Fat: 2g; Monounsaturated Fat: 2g; Cholesterol: 65mg; Sodium: 291mg; Carbohydrates: 58g; Fiber: 10g; Sugars: 8g; Protein: 34g

SUBSTITUTION TIP: Not a fan of gluten-free pasta? Want additional protein? Use quinoa in place of the spaghetti.

SPICY WHITE CHICKEN CHILI

Prep time: 15 minutes / Cook time: 4 hours on high or 8 hours on low

There's nothing like a recipe with the perfect balance of flavor, lean protein, high-fiber beans, and vegetables. I did mention flavor, right? Turn up the heat with this flavor-packed white chili.

Serves 7

1½ pounds boneless, skinless chicken breasts

4 cups Chicken Stock (page 25) or Savory Vegetable Broth (page 24)

2 (14-ounce) cans no-salt-added cannellini beans, drained and rinsed

2 cups frozen corn

2 green bell peppers, chopped

3 jalapeño peppers, seeded, membranes removed, minced

1 onion, chopped

1 (4-ounce) can diced green chiles

4 garlic cloves, minced

2 teaspoons ground cumin

1 teaspoon chili powder

1 teaspoon dried oregano

½ teaspoon salt

¼ teaspoon cayenne pepper

¼ cup yellow cornmeal

¼ cup fat-free or low-fat milk, or plant-based milk

1 cup chopped cilantro

1 lime, cut into wedges

1. Place the chicken, stock, beans, corn, bell peppers, jalapeños, onion, chiles, garlic, cumin, chili powder, oregano, salt, and cayenne pepper in a 6-quart slow cooker. Cover and cook on high for 4 hours or on low for 8 hours.

2. Just prior to serving, mix together the cornmeal and milk in a small bowl. Stir this into the slow cooker and allow the sauce to thicken slightly, about 5 minutes.

3. Serve hot, topped with the cilantro and a squeeze of lime juice.

Per Serving (2 cups): Calories: 319; Total Fat: 4g; Saturated Fat: 1g; Trans Fat: 0g; Polyunsaturated Fat: 1g; Monounsaturated Fat: 2g; Cholesterol: 56mg; Sodium: 335mg; Carbohydrates: 40g; Fiber: 8g; Sugars: 6g; Protein: 32g

NUTRITION HIGHLIGHT: Rather than adding more salt to recipes, boost the flavor with fresh herbs and citrus. A sprinkling of cilantro and a squeeze of lime juice accentuate the flavors of this recipe in a heart-healthy way.

NO-FUSS TURKEY BREAST

Prep time: 15 minutes / Cook time: 7 to 8 hours on low

This slow cooker turkey breast recipe is perfect for smaller get-togethers and doesn't heat up your house for hours like using your oven does. Slow cooking the turkey is an easy, safe, and tasty way to cook your turkey to juicy perfection.

Serves 8

1 (4- to 5-pound) bone-in turkey breast, skin removed, thawed (if frozen)

1 tablespoon extra-virgin olive oil

2 teaspoons dried thyme

1 teaspoon paprika

1 teaspoon dried garlic

Freshly ground black pepper

Nonstick cooking spray

2 cups Brussels sprouts, halved

2 onions, cut into large chunks, divided

4 celery ribs, cut into 3-inch lengths

12 baby carrots

1 cup Turkey Stock (page 26) or low-sodium turkey broth

4 or 5 fresh thyme sprigs (optional)

1. Brush the turkey with the olive oil.

2. In a small bowl, mix together the dried thyme, paprika, garlic, and black pepper. Rub the mixture all over the turkey.

3. Spray a 6-quart slow cooker with the cooking spray. Add the Brussels sprouts, chunks of 1 onion, celery, and carrots, to the slow cooker. Pour the broth over the vegetables. Place the turkey breast on top of the vegetables, making sure it does not touch the bottom of the slow cooker. Cover the turkey with the chunks of the second onion and the fresh thyme (if using).

4. Cover and cook on low for 7 to 8 hours, or until the turkey's internal temperature reaches 165°F.

5. Let the turkey rest for 10 minutes before carving. Serve hot, with fresh Cranberry Sauce (page 23) and your favorite fixings.

Per Serving (1 cup): Calories: 367; Total Fat: 10g; Saturated Fat: 3g; Trans Fat: 0g; Polyunsaturated Fat: 0g; Monounsaturated Fat: 1g; Cholesterol: 147mg; Sodium: 380mg; Carbohydrates: 9g; Fiber: 2g; Sugars: 2g; Protein: 60g

COOKING TIP: It is not safe to thaw a turkey breast in the slow cooker. To safely thaw a turkey, put it in the refrigerator and allow 24 hours for a 4- to 5-pound turkey breast.

MINI TURKEY-VEGGIE MEATBALLS

Prep time: 15 minutes / Cook time: 6 to 7 hours on low

These simple turkey-veggie meatballs are easy to make ahead of time and are freezer-friendly. The shredded zucchini and carrots keep the lean ground turkey nice and moist while sneaking in fiber- and nutrient-rich vegetables. Mix and match your favorite vegetables and herbs, and you will never grow tired of these healthy high-protein meatballs that are perfect for busy weeknights.

Serves 8

2 pounds 93% lean ground turkey breast

1 cup shredded zucchini

1 cup finely shredded carrots

½ cup quick oats

2 garlic cloves, minced

1 large egg, lightly beaten

2 tablespoons extra-virgin olive oil, divided

¼ cup chopped flat leaf parsley

Freshly ground black pepper

4 shallots, minced

2 (28-ounce) cans no-salt-diced tomatoes, divided

1. Combine the turkey, zucchini, carrots, oats, garlic, egg, 1 tablespoon olive oil, parsley, and black pepper in a large bowl. Roll the mixture into 30 (or more) mini meatballs, each about the size of a golf ball, and place on a baking sheet.

2. Optional step: Heat the remaining 1 tablespoon of olive oil in a large nonstick skillet over medium-high heat. Working in batches if needed, add the meatballs about 1 inch apart, searing them on the top and bottom until golden, about 1 minute per side.

3. Put the shallots and 1 can of tomatoes in the slow cooker. Add the meatballs one at a time, stacking them if necessary. Cover the meatballs with the remaining can of tomatoes. Cook on low for 6 to 7 hours, until the meatballs are cooked through.

4. Serve hot over vegetable noodles or pasta, or with just a simple green salad, if desired.

Per Serving (3 to 4 mini meatballs): Calories: 277; Total Fat: 12g; Saturated Fat: 3g; Trans Fat: 0g; Polyunsaturated Fat: 1g; Monounsaturated Fat: 3g; Cholesterol: 103mg; Sodium: 132mg; Carbohydrates: 16g; Fiber: 3g; Sugars: 1g; Protein: 25g

MAKE-AHEAD: Browning the meatballs in the skillet gives them an even deeper flavor. You can brown the meatballs the day before you plan to cook them and then refrigerate until ready to use. You could also freeze them once browned, but be sure to allow them to thaw overnight in the refrigerator before you put them in the slow cooker.

TURKEY AND MUSHROOM WILD RICE CASSEROLE

Prep time: 15 minutes / Cook time: 7 to 8 hours on low

This herbed turkey and mushroom wild rice casserole uses a simple homemade condensed creamed soup to keep the sodium in check and add savory flavor without unhealthy additives. A garnish of crunchy almonds and chopped green onions finishes this comforting casserole-like dish.

Serves 8

Nonstick cooking spray

1 cup cold low-fat or fat-free milk, or plant-based milk

3 tablespoons extra-virgin olive oil

3 tablespoons cornstarch

6 cups Turkey Stock (page 26) or low-sodium turkey broth, divided

2 pounds turkey breast tenderloin, cut into ¾-inch pieces

2 cups wild rice, rinsed and drained

1 onion, chopped

1 cup sliced carrot

1 cup sliced celery

1 cup sliced button mushrooms

1 teaspoon dried tarragon

¼ teaspoon freshly ground black pepper

½ cup sliced almonds

½ cup chopped scallions, for garnish (optional)

1. Spray the inside of a 6-quart slow cooker with the cooking spray.

2. In a small bowl, whisk together the cold milk, olive oil, and cornstarch. Add 1 cup of broth and whisk to combine. Pour this mixture into the slow cooker.

3. Add the turkey, rice, onion, carrot, celery, mushrooms, tarragon, and black pepper to the slow cooker. Pour in the remaining 5 cups of broth and stir to combine. Cover and cook on low for 7 to 8 hours, until vegetables are tender, the rice has absorbed the liquid, and the turkey is cooked through.

4. Serve hot, garnished with the sliced almonds and scallions, if using.

Per Serving (1½ cups): Calories: 420; Total Fat: 9g; Saturated Fat: 1g; Trans Fat: 0g; Polyunsaturated Fat: 1g; Monounsaturated Fat: 4g; Cholesterol: 70mg; Sodium: 158mg; Carbohydrates: 42g; Fiber: 4g; Sugars: 2g; Protein: 40g

COOKING TIP: Use this basic creamed soup substitute as a healthier alternative to canned in all of your favorite recipes. To make on the stove top: Heat the oil, then stir in the cornstarch and seasonings and cook until bubbly. Add the turkey stock slowly, stirring with a wire whisk to prevent clumps, and cook until thick.

ASIAN TURKEY LETTUCE WRAPS

Prep time: 10 minutes / Cook time: 6 to 7 hours on low

This light and flavorful Asian-inspired meal is simple to prep and full of satisfying protein and fiber-rich vegetables. The crunchy lettuce, carrots, and cabbage go well with the seasoned slow-cooked turkey. Top with your favorite hot sauce and serve with brown rice, if desired.

Serves 8

- 2 pounds 93% lean ground turkey breast meat
- 1 (8-ounce) can water chestnuts, drained and sliced
- 2 red bell peppers, chopped
- 1 onion, finely chopped
- 1 cup frozen, shelled edamame
- 4 garlic cloves, minced
- 2 tablespoons low-sodium tamari
- 2 tablespoons rice wine vinegar
- 1 tablespoon grated fresh ginger
- 2 teaspoons sesame oil
- 1 teaspoon ground coriander
- 1 head romaine lettuce leaves
- 1 cup finely shredded carrot
- 1 cup finely shredded cabbage
- 4 tablespoons sesame seeds

1. Crumble the ground turkey into a 6-quart slow cooker. Add the water chestnuts, bell peppers, onion, edamame, garlic, tamari, vinegar, ginger, sesame oil, and coriander and stir to combine. Cover and cook on low for 6 to 7 hours.

2. Wrap the meat mixture evenly in the lettuce leaves and top with the carrots, cabbage, and sesame seeds.

Per Serving (2 wraps with ½ cup turkey mixture): Calories: 249; Total Fat: 12g; Saturated Fat: 4g; Trans Fat: 0g; Polyunsaturated Fat: 3g; Monounsaturated Fat: 4g; Cholesterol: 80mg; Sodium: 240mg; Carbohydrates: 10g; Fiber: 3g; Sugars: 2g; Protein: 26g

COOKING TIP: You can customize the spices in this recipe to your liking. Some good choices include Chinese five-spice powder, chili powder, Chinese cinnamon, cloves, and lemongrass.

TUSCAN TURKEY, WHITE BEANS, AND ASPARAGUS

Prep time: 15 minutes, plus overnight to soak / Cook time: 7 to 8 hours on low,
plus 15 to 20 minutes on high

Food from the Tuscan region of Italy is characterized by its simplicity. It is prepared without heavy sauces or elaborate seasonings. With those principles in mind, this simple, yet flavorful, garlicky bean and turkey recipe uses just a handful of ingredients to create a nourishing and filling meal.

Serves 8

Nonstick cooking spray

1 pound dried cannellini beans, soaked overnight and drained

3 cups Turkey Stock (page 26) or low-sodium turkey stock

3 tablespoons extra-virgin olive oil

6 garlic cloves, minced

1 teaspoon dried sage

1 teaspoon dried rosemary

Freshly ground black pepper

2 pounds turkey thighs, skin removed

3 cups chopped asparagus

1. Spray a 6-quart slow cooker with the cooking spray. Put the beans in the slow cooker and add the broth.

2. In a small bowl, stir together the olive oil, garlic, sage, rosemary, and black pepper. Press this mixture firmly into the turkey thighs. Place the turkey on top of the beans in the slow cooker. Cover and cook on low for 7 to 8 hours, until the beans are tender and the turkey reaches an internal temperature of 165°F.

3. Remove the turkey from the slow cooker and increase the heat to high. Add the asparagus and cook for 15 to 20 minutes, or until the asparagus is bright green and crisp tender.

4. While the asparagus is cooking, remove the turkey meat from the bones. To serve, ladle the bean and asparagus mixture into bowls and top with the turkey meat.

Per Serving (½ cup turkey meat with 1 cup vegetables):
Calories: 326; Total Fat: 12g; Saturated Fat: 1g; Trans Fat: 0g; Polyunsaturated Fat: 1g; Monounsaturated Fat: 4g; Cholesterol: 70mg; Sodium: 72mg; Carbohydrates: 39g; Fiber: 21g; Sugars: 2g; Protein: 26g

NUTRITIONAL HIGHLIGHT: Asparagus has an impressive array of nutritional benefits. A very-low-calorie food, this green veggie is good source of B vitamins and minerals, and acts as a natural diuretic, which is helpful for people with high blood pressure.

SWEET-AND-SOUR TURKEY LEGS AND PEPPERS

Prep time: 10 minutes / Cook time: 7 to 8 hours on low

Turkey legs get an exotic island flavor from a simple, homemade sweet-and-sour sauce that keeps the meat moist during the slow-cooking process. Red bell peppers, garlic, and shallots add extra flavor so that all you need to complete the meal is your favorite grain or potato and green veggie.

Serves 6

Nonstick cooking spray

6 turkey legs, skin removed

2 red bell peppers, chopped

4 shallots, chopped

½ cup Homemade Ketchup (page 20)

⅓ cup cider vinegar

2 tablespoons brown sugar

1 tablespoon low-sodium soy sauce

¼ teaspoon dried mustard

¼ teaspoon dried onion powder

4 garlic cloves, minced

1 (8-ounce) can crushed pineapple, drained

1. Spray the inside of a 6-quart slow cooker with the cooking spray. Place the turkey legs in the slow cooker. Add the bell peppers and shallots.

2. In a small bowl, whisk together the ketchup, vinegar, brown sugar, soy sauce, dried mustard, onion powder, garlic, and pineapple. Spoon this over the turkey legs and turn to coat the legs well.

3. Cover and cook on low for 7 to 8 hours, until the turkey is cooked through and the peppers are tender.

4. Serve hot.

Per Serving (1 leg plus ⅓ cup sauce): Calories: 208; Total Fat: 3g; Saturated Fat: 1g; Trans Fat: 0g; Polyunsaturated Fat: 1g; Monounsaturated Fat: 1g; Cholesterol: 86mg; Sodium: 169mg; Carbohydrates: 24g; Fiber: 1g; Sugars: 16g; Protein: 21g

NUTRITIONAL HIGHLIGHT: Shallots are petite members of the Allium plant genus, which also includes onion and garlic. And just like onions and garlic, shallots are known to have strong heart-health, immunity-enhancing, and anti-cancer effects. You can use shallots wherever you would use onions.

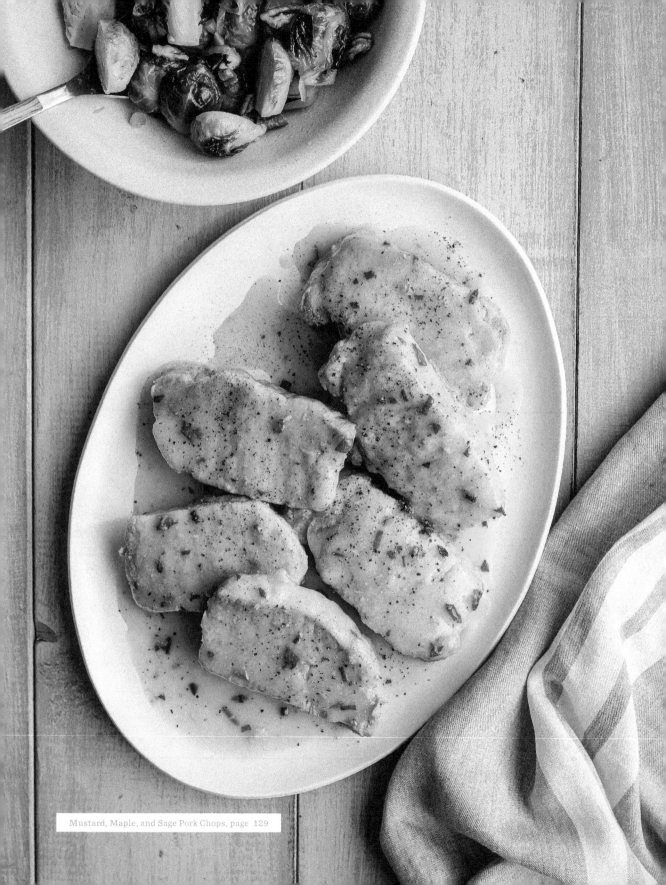

Mustard, Maple, and Sage Pork Chops, page 129

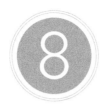

Beef, Pork, and Lamb Mains

BEEF AND BROCCOLI

Prep time: 10 minutes / Cook time: 6 to 7 hours on low

American Chinese food is generally very high in sodium. This recipe is even easier than picking up Chinese takeout, plus it is much healthier with its lower-sodium homemade sauce. This meal is as flavorful and tasty as takeout and can be on the table in minutes—a perfect ending to a long workday.

Serves 6

1 cup Beef Stock (page 27) or low-sodium beef broth

4 garlic cloves, minced

¼ cup low-sodium soy sauce

¼ cup balsamic vinegar

¼ cup honey

1 tablespoon sesame oil

1 teaspoon grated fresh ginger

¼ teaspoon red pepper flakes

2 pounds flank steak, cut into thin strips

2 tablespoons cornstarch

4 cups frozen broccoli florets

2 red bell peppers, cut into thin strips

1. In a small bowl, whisk together the stock, garlic, soy sauce, vinegar, honey, sesame oil, ginger, and red pepper flakes.

2. Place the beef into a 6-quart slow cooker. Add the sauce mixture and stir to combine. Cover and cook on low for 6 to 7 hours, until the meat is cooked through and tender.

3. About 30 minutes before serving, stir in the cornstarch. Then add the broccoli and peppers and continue cooking until the vegetables are tender and the sauce has thickened.

4. Serve hot over rice with additional red pepper flakes and a sprinkle of sesame seeds, if desired.

Per Serving (1½ cups): Calories: 353; Total Fat: 13g; Saturated Fat: 5g; Trans Fat: 0g; Polyunsaturated Fat: 2g; Monounsaturated Fat: 6g; Cholesterol: 53mg; Sodium: 505mg; Carbohydrates: 23g; Fiber: 2g; Sugars: 14g; Protein: 35g

COOKING TIP: For easier cleanup, try using a slow cooker liner. A liner can work for any recipe in this book.

PORK ROAST WITH APPLES, ROOT VEGETABLES, AND ROSEMARY

Prep time: 10 minutes / Cook time: 8 hours on low

Pork and apples are a classic combination. This recipe combines the sweet flavors of apples with delicious root vegetables and savory pork. Fragrant rosemary enhances the flavors in this simple meal that includes lean protein, and fiber- and nutrient-rich fruit and vegetables.

Serves 8

3 apples, thickly sliced (peeling is optional)

2 cups peeled and cubed sweet potato

4 large carrots, cut into 1-inch pieces

1 cup parsnips, chopped

1 Vidalia onion, sliced

1 (4-pound) boneless pork loin roast

8 fresh rosemary sprigs

1 cup Beef Stock (page 27) or low-sodium beef broth

1. Line the bottom of a 6-quart slow cooker with half of the apples, sweet potato, carrots, parsnips, and onion. Place the pork on top of the vegetables. Lay the rosemary on top of the pork and cover with the remaining apples and vegetables. Pour the stock over the pork and vegetables.

2. Cover and cook on low for 8 hours, or until the pork reaches an internal temperature of 160°F.

3. Remove the pork from the slow cooker and allow it to rest for 3 minutes. Slice and serve with the apples and vegetables.

Per Serving (2¼ cups): Calories: 398; Total Fat: 9g; Saturated Fat: 3g; Trans Fat: 0g; Polyunsaturated Fat: 1g; Monounsaturated Fat: 4g; Cholesterol: 140mg; Sodium: 210mg; Carbohydrates: 24g; Fiber: 4g; Sugars: 12g; Protein: 52g

COOKING TIP: To safely cook pork chops, roasts, and tenderloins the National Pork Board recommends cooking to an internal temperature between 145°F (medium rare) and 160°F (medium), followed by a 3-minute rest before serving.

CITRUSY MEXICAN PULLED PORK

Prep time: 15 minutes / Cook time: 4 hours on high or 8 hours on low

Traditional carnitas is made with pork shoulder, which is extremely high in saturated fat. It is also traditionally fried in some oil before serving, resulting in an even higher fat content. Here, a spicy, bold rub and fragrant citrus juice is used to flavor the pork loin. This Mexican pulled pork is healthy, but still packed with flavor.

Serves 6

1 tablespoon dried oregano

2 teaspoons ground cumin

2 teaspoons garlic powder

2 teaspoons onion powder

¼ teaspoon cayenne pepper

2 pounds boneless pork loin, trimmed of fat

½ onion, chopped

3 garlic cloves, minced

1 jalapeño pepper, seeded and chopped

Juice of 1 lime

Juice of 1 orange

1. Combine the oregano, cumin, garlic powder, onion powder, and cayenne in a small bowl. Rub this mixture over the entire surface of the pork loin. Place the pork into a 4- to 6-quart slow cooker.

2. Top the pork with the onion, minced garlic, jalapeño, lime juice, and orange juice. Cover and cook on high for 4 hours or on low for 8 hours.

3. Remove the pork and shred it using two forks. Return the shredded pork to the slow cooker to soak up the liquid and to keep hot before serving.

Per Serving (5 ounces): Calories: 243; Total Fat: 11g; Saturated Fat: 4g; Trans Fat: 0g; Polyunsaturated Fat: 1g; Monounsaturated Fat: 5g; Cholesterol: 73mg; Sodium: 150mg; Carbohydrates: 7g; Fiber: 2g; Sugars: 3g; Protein: 29g

MAKE-AHEAD: Consider doubling this recipe so you'll have leftovers to freeze. Pulled pork freezes beautifully and makes future meals quick and easy.

MUSTARD, MAPLE, AND SAGE PORK CHOPS

Prep time: 5 minutes / Cook time: 4 hours on high or 7 to 8 hours on low

This trio of flavors—maple, mustard, and sage—is an absolute gem and perfect on pork. This sauce is finger-licking good and fat-free: proof positive that heart-healthy food doesn't have to be bland and boring.

Serves 6

5 tablespoons apple
    cider vinegar

4 tablespoons Dijon mustard

3 tablespoons pure maple syrup

2 tablespoons extra-virgin
    olive oil

1 tablespoon fresh sage, minced

½ teaspoon freshly ground
    black pepper

6 (5-ounce) boneless pork chops

1 tablespoon cornstarch

2 tablespoons water

1. In the bottom of a 4- to 6-quart slow cooker, whisk together the vinegar, mustard, maple syrup, olive oil, sage, and black pepper. Add the pork chops and flip them to coat in the mustard mixture.

2. Cover and cook on high for 4 hours or on low for 7 to 8 hours. Transfer the pork chops to a plate and cover them with aluminum foil; set aside.

3. If you cooked the pork on high heat, reduce the heat to low. In a small bowl, whisk together the cornstarch and water until smooth. Whisk this into the sauce in the slow cooker until smooth. Cover and allow the sauce to thicken for about 5 minutes. Add pork chops back to the slow cooker to warm through.

4. Serve the pork chops hot, topped with the sauce.

Per Serving (1 prepared chop): Calories: 255; Total Fat: 11g; Saturated Fat: 3g; Trans Fat: 0g; Polyunsaturated Fat: 1g; Monounsaturated Fat: 3g; Cholesterol: 69mg; Sodium: 331mg; Carbohydrates: 8g; Fiber: 0g; Sugars: 7g; Protein: 26g

VARIATION TIP: Swap in chicken or pork loin in place of the pork chops. Both are lean and showcase this perfect combination of flavors in a heart-healthy way.

TEX-MEX SLOPPY JOES

Prep time: 10 minutes / Cook time: 6 to 8 hours on low

Most sloppy Joe mixes are *very* high in sodium. This slow cooker version is quick to prep and made with an easy-to-assemble homemade sauce with much less salt. A mix of lean ground pork and beef plus a cup of shredded zucchini gives this recipe a nutrition boost while sneaking in some extra vegetables. Slow cooking makes a sauce with a deeper, richer flavor. This is a great way to feed a crowd!

Serves 8

1½ pounds 93% lean
    ground beef

1½ pounds lean ground pork

1½ cups Homemade
    Ketchup (page 20)

1 (8-ounce) can no-salt-
    added tomato sauce

1 medium onion, finely chopped

1 medium bell pepper
    (any color), diced

1 cup shredded zucchini

4 garlic cloves, minced

2 tablespoons honey

2 tablespoons yellow mustard

1 tablespoon
    Worcestershire sauce

1 tablespoon chili powder

1. Combine all the ingredients in a 6-quart slow cooker, making sure to break up the beef and pork. Cover and cook on low for 6 to 8 hours.

2. Serve immediately. The sloppy Joe mixture can be served on whole-wheat buns or wrapped in lettuce leaves, if desired.

Per Serving (1 cup): Calories: 393; Total Fat: 10g; Saturated Fat: 4g; Trans Fat: 0g; Polyunsaturated Fat: 2g; Monounsaturated Fat: 4g; Cholesterol: 97mg; Sodium: 191mg; Carbohydrates: 29g; Fiber: 1g; Sugars: 19g; Protein: 37g

VARIATION TIP: Although many slow cooker sloppy Joe recipes suggest browning the meat before adding it to the slow cooker, this step isn't essential, because of the long cooking time. However, if you have the time, you can deepen the flavor by simply cooking the meat, onion, and garlic in a large skillet until browned. Drain off the fat and add to the slow cooker.

KOREAN BEEF TACOS

Prep time: 10 minutes / Cook time: 8 to 10 hours on low

This taco recipe combines spicy, sweet, and savory fillings and is super easy to make at home with all of the comfort and heartiness of authentic Korean food.

Serves 8

1 large red onion, sliced thin

3 pounds flank steak, trimmed of fat

⅓ cup honey

¼ cup rice wine vinegar

4 garlic cloves, minced

1 jalapeño pepper, seeded and finely diced

3 tablespoons low-sodium soy sauce or tamari

2 tablespoons minced fresh ginger

1 tablespoon sesame oil

16 (6-inch) corn tortillas

2 cups finely shredded cabbage, for garnish

1 cup chopped fresh cilantro, for garnish

Sriracha sauce, for garnish

1. Place the onion on the bottom of a 6-quart slow cooker. Add the steak, honey, vinegar, garlic, jalapeño, soy sauce, ginger, and sesame oil. Cover and cook on low for 8 to 10 hours.

2. Shred the beef with a pair of forks and stir it into the liquid in the slow cooker.

3. Serve the beef in the corn tortillas. If desired, garnish with shredded cabbage, cilantro, and sriracha sauce.

Per Serving (2 tacos): Calories: 335; Total Fat: 14g; Saturated Fat: 5g; Trans Fat: 0g; Polyunsaturated Fat: 2g; Monounsaturated Fat: 6g; Cholesterol: 60mg; Sodium: 300mg; Carbohydrates: 14g; Fiber: 0g; Sugars: 13g; Protein: 37g

COOKING TIP: Korean cooking is characterized by its full flavor and spicy kick from the gochujang, which is a thick, fermented, hot pepper paste. For a more authentic Korean flavor, add 1 tablespoon garlic chili sauce or 1 tablespoon gochujang paste, which you can find in an Asian specialty market or online.

STUFFED CABBAGE CASSEROLE

Prep time: 10 minutes / Cook time: 7 to 8 hours on low

Cabbage casserole is so much easier and quicker to prepare than making the rolls individually, and it is just as delicious. A simple ground beef mixture is topped with cabbage and tomatoes, and cooked with fiber-rich brown rice. The combination can't be beat for a filling, tasty, and nutritious comfort meal.

Serves 8

1 tablespoon extra-virgin olive oil

1½ pounds 93% lean ground beef

1 onion, chopped

4 garlic cloves, minced

Nonstick cooking spray

1½ cups brown rice

1 medium head green cabbage, cored and chopped (about 6 cups)

2 cups Rustic Marinara Sauce (page 16)

1 (14.5-ounce) can no-salt-added diced tomatoes

1 cup Spicy Salsa (page 19)

1 cup Beef Stock (page 27) or low-sodium beef broth

1 bell pepper (any color), chopped

1 teaspoon smoked paprika

1 teaspoon dried thyme

1. Optional step: In a large skillet over medium-high heat, add the olive oil. Add the ground beef, onion, and garlic and cook until the beef is browned, 7 to 10 minutes.

2. Spray the inside of a 6-quart slow cooker with the cooking spray. Place the rice in the bottom of the slow cooker followed by half of the cabbage. Add the beef and vegetables over the cabbage layer (using a slotted spoon if these ingredients were browned ahead of time).

3. Add the remaining cabbage along with the marinara, tomatoes, salsa, stock, bell pepper, paprika, and thyme (the cooker may seem too full, but the cabbage will shrink during cooking). Cover and cook on low for 7 to 8 hours, until the rice is cooked and the vegetables are tender.

4. Serve hot.

Per Serving (2 cups): Calories: 365; Total Fat: 8g; Saturated Fat: 3g; Trans Fat: 0g; Polyunsaturated Fat: 1g; Monounsaturated Fat: 3g; Cholesterol: 48mg; Sodium: 318mg; Carbohydrates: 45g; Fiber: 6g; Sugars: 7g; Protein: 23g

NUTRITIONAL HIGHLIGHT: Many people are put off by the strong taste of cabbage, but this vegetable is a powerhouse of nutrition. Cabbage is an excellent source of vitamins K, C, and B6. It is also a very good source of fiber and heart-healthy potassium, plus it is very low in calories.

SPRING BEEF BOURGUIGNON

Prep time: 15 minutes / Cook time: 7 to 8 hours on low

This delicious beef bourguignon (meaning cooked in a red wine sauce) is a heart-healthy variation of the classic French recipe. With spring vegetables, including asparagus and leeks, along with the traditional potatoes and carrots, this hearty dish is packed with protein and fiber for a satisfying meal. It puts an elegant spin on comfort food.

Serves 8

1½ pounds lean beef roast, cut into bite-size cubes

2 tablespoons all-purpose flour

2 tablespoons extra-virgin olive oil, divided

4 garlic cloves, minced

2 cups halved button mushrooms

2 leeks, white and light green parts, sliced thinly

2 carrots, sliced thinly

1½ cups dry red wine

1½ cups Beef Stock (page 27) or low-sodium beef broth

1 pound small red potatoes

2 teaspoons dried thyme

1 teaspoon dried rosemary

2 cups chopped asparagus

1. Toss the beef cubes with the flour and 1 tablespoon olive oil.

2. Optional step: Heat a large skillet over medium-high heat. (Do not add oil.) Add the beef cubes and cook, stirring once or twice until seared and browned on several sides and no longer pink on the inside, 7 to 8 minutes. Transfer the beef to the slow cooker. Return the skillet to the heat, add the remaining 1 tablespoon of oil. Add the garlic, mushrooms, leeks, and carrots and cook until the vegetables begin to soften, 3 to 5 minutes. Transfer the vegetables to the slow cooker. If not browning these ingredients, just put them all directly into the slow cooker.

3. Add the wine, stock (or broth), potatoes, thyme, and rosemary to the slow cooker. Cover and cook on low for 7 to 8 hours. In the last 30 minutes, add the asparagus and continue cooking until crisp tender.

4. Serve hot.

Per Serving (1¾ cups): Calories: 292; Total Fat: 12g; Saturated Fat: 5g; Trans Fat: 0g; Polyunsaturated Fat: 2g; Monounsaturated Fat: 4g; Cholesterol: 41mg; Sodium: 274mg; Carbohydrates: 17g; Fiber: 3g; Sugars: 3g; Protein: 20g

COOKING TIP: If you like your stew thicker, mix 1 to 2 additional tablespoons of flour into the beef stock before adding it to the slow cooker. To make this recipe gluten-free, simply swap the flour for cornstarch.

TANGY ITALIAN BEEF SANDWICHES

Prep time: 5 minutes / Cook time: 8 hours on low

This beef roast tenderizes to perfection in the slow cooker with help from the slightly acidic and considerably tangy pepperoncini peppers. It's simple yet flavorful and everything you can hope for in a heart-healthy sandwich.

Serves 8

4 pounds eye of round boneless roast, trimmed of fat

1 (16-ounce) jar pepperoncini, with all but ¼ cup of their liquid

8 French sub buns, sliced

1. Place the beef roast in a 6-quart slow cooker. Top it with the pepperoncini and the liquid. Cover and cook on low for 8 hours.

2. Shred the meat using two forks and return it to the slow cooker.

3. Drizzle some of the accumulated juices over the inside portion of the bun before filling with the shredded beef. Serve immediately.

Per Serving (6 ounces beef plus a bun): Calories: 463; Total Fat: 10g; Saturated Fat: 3g; Trans Fat: 0g; Polyunsaturated Fat: 0g; Monounsaturated Fat: 0g; Cholesterol: 109mg; Sodium: 425mg; Carbohydrates: 35g; Fiber: 1g; Sugars: 2g; Protein: 59g

> SUBSTITUTION TIP: Swap in a gluten-free bun to make this meal gluten-free. Or pump up the fiber content by using a whole-wheat sub bun.

ITALIAN PORK WITH BEANS AND GREENS

Prep time: 10 minutes / Cook time: 8 to 9 hours on low

This Italian pork shoulder recipe is packed so full of flavor your family won't even notice they are eating nutritious fiber-rich beans and dark leafy greens. The slow cooking makes the pork fork-tender and the vegetables just melt in your mouth.

Serves 8

Nonstick cooking spray

2 pounds pork shoulder, visible fat removed

1 teaspoon dried basil

1 teaspoon dried oregano

1 onion, chopped

2 medium carrots, sliced

4 garlic cloves, minced

1 cup Chicken Stock (page 25) or low-sodium chicken broth

1 (14.5-ounce) can no-salt-added diced tomatoes

1 (15-ounce) can cannellini beans, drained and rinsed

2 cups chopped fresh green beans

2 cups chopped spinach

1. Spray the inside of a 6-quart slow cooker with the cooking spray. Add the pork and sprinkle it with the basil and oregano. Add the onion, carrots, and garlic and pour in the stock and tomatoes. Cover and cook on low for 7 to 8 hours.

2. Break up the meat into large chunks. Add the cannellini beans, green beans, and spinach. Cover and continue cooking for 1 hour more, until the vegetables are tender and the internal temperature of the pork reaches 160°F.

3. Serve hot, with potatoes or rice if desired.

Per Serving (1⅔ cups): Calories: 320; Total Fat: 10g; Saturated Fat: 4g; Trans Fat: 0g; Polyunsaturated Fat: 1g; Monounsaturated Fat: 5g; Cholesterol: 96mg; Sodium: 207mg; Carbohydrates: 16g; Fiber: 4g; Sugars: 2g; Protein: 38g

NUTRITIONAL HIGHLIGHT: Spinach is an excellent source of important vitamins, minerals, and health-promoting antioxidants. This green veggie is extremely versatile, very low in calories, and a good source of fiber.

LAMB ROAST WITH ROOT VEGETABLES

Prep time: 10 minutes / Cook time: 7 to 8 hours on low

This elegant meal tastes as good as it looks and requires very little prep work or cleanup. Slow cooking the lamb with rosemary, garlic, and winter vegetables creates a melt-in-your-mouth flavorful meal full of lean protein and nutrient-rich vegetables.

Serves 8

4 pounds cubed lamb meat

4 garlic cloves, minced

2 or 3 fresh rosemary sprigs

Nonstick cooking spray

2 teaspoons freshly ground black pepper

6 carrots, sliced

4 beets, peeled and cut into wedges

2 medium parsnips, peeled and sliced

2 medium sweet potatoes, peeled and cut into wedges

2 medium turnips, peeled and cut into wedges

2 medium Yukon gold potatoes, cut into wedges

2 cups Chicken Stock (page 25) or low-sodium chicken broth

1. Make incisions in roast and press in the garlic and rosemary.

2. Lightly coat the bowl of a 6-quart slow cooker with the cooking spray. Place the lamb into the slow cooker and sprinkle it with the black pepper. Place any loose rosemary leaves in the slow cooker, too.

3. Arrange the carrots, beets, parsnips, sweet potatoes, turnips, and potatoes around the meat. Pour in the stock. Cover and cook on low for 7 to 8 hours, until the vegetables are tender and the meat reaches an internal temperature of 160°F.

4. Remove the roast and let rest for 5 to 10 minutes before slicing and serving.

Per Serving (2 cups): Calories: 459; Total Fat: 12g; Saturated Fat: 4g; Trans Fat: 0g; Polyunsaturated Fat: 2g; Monounsaturated Fat: 5g; Cholesterol: 147mg; Sodium: 257mg; Carbohydrates: 34g; Fiber: 6g; Sugars: 11g; Protein: 49g

NUTRITIONAL HIGHLIGHT: According to the American Lamb Board, 40 percent of the fat in lean cuts of lamb is monounsaturated fat, the same type of fat found in olive oil. Lamb is also an excellent source of vitamin B12, niacin, zinc, and selenium.

BEEF AND VEGETABLE STEW

Prep time: 10 minutes / Cook time: 6 to 8 hours on low

This recipe has all of the traditional flavors of Grandma's beef stew complete with a tasty sauce and hearty and chunky vegetables. With melt-in-your-mouth beef, this recipe is an absolute delight the whole family will love.

Serves 6

1 tablespoon extra-virgin olive oil (optional)

2 pounds beef stew meat, cubed

4 cups Beef Stock (page 27) or low-sodium beef broth

1 (14-ounce) can no-salt-added diced tomatoes

½ pound baby potatoes, quartered

½ pound parsnips, peeled and cubed

4 medium carrots, chopped

2 cups green beans, fresh or frozen

1 medium onion, diced

2 celery stalks, diced

2 garlic cloves, minced

2 teaspoons dried thyme

3 tablespoons cold water

2 tablespoons cornstarch

1. Optional step: Heat the oil in a large nonstick skillet over medium-high heat. Add the beef and cook until browned on all sides, 2 to 3 minutes. (If you choose not to brown the meat first, the olive oil does not need to be added to the slow cooker.)

2. Add the beef, stock, tomatoes, potatoes, parsnips, carrots, green beans, onion, celery, garlic, and thyme to a 6-quart slow cooker. Cover and cook on low for 6 to 8 hours.

3. With 30 minutes left to cook, combine the cold water and cornstarch, stirring until the cornstarch is dissolved. Stir this into the stew. Turn the slow cooker to the high setting and continue cooking until the stew is thickened.

4. Serve hot.

Per Serving (2 cups): Calories: 354; Total Fat: 9g; Saturated Fat: 3g; Trans Fat: 0g; Polyunsaturated Fat: 2g; Monounsaturated Fat: 4g; Cholesterol: 100mg; Sodium: 445mg; Carbohydrates: 26g; Fiber: 5g; Sugars: 7g; Protein: 38g

> **MAKE-AHEAD:** Chop the parsnips, carrots, celery, and green beans the day before and put them in a resealable bag and refrigerate. Chop the potatoes and onions and refrigerate them in a separate resealable bag. Last, cut the beef into chunks and place them in their own resealable bag and refrigerate.

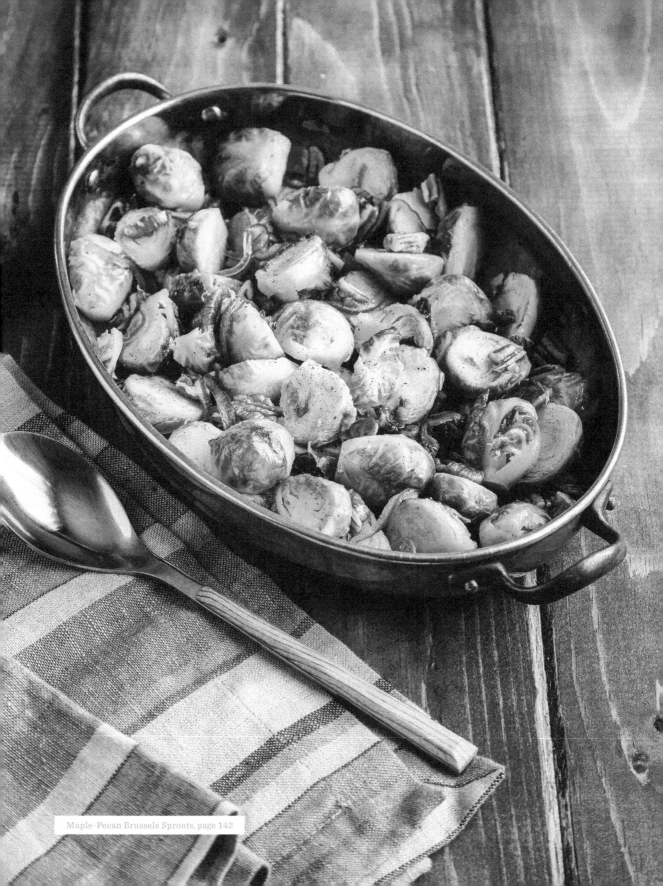

Maple-Pecan Brussels Sprouts, page 142

9

Sides

CREAMY SPICED MASHED CAULIFLOWER

Prep time: 10 minutes / Cook time: 6 hours on low

Mashed cauliflower is a fantastic low-calorie and low-carb alternative to mashed pota-toes. Preparing this dish in the slow cooker is a breeze. This variation, which goes great with curries, uses Indian spices, but feel free to use more traditional herbs. Its beauty is that it can be customized to your taste.

Serves 6

1 large head cauliflower, cut into medium-size florets (about 8 cups)

6 garlic cloves, minced

4 cups Savory Vegetable Broth (page 24) or low-sodium vegetable broth

1 to 2 cups water

2 tablespoons extra-virgin olive oil

⅓ cup plain nonfat Greek yogurt

1 teaspoon ground turmeric

1 teaspoon curry powder

½ teaspoon ground ginger

1. Put the cauliflower in a 6-quart slow cooker and top it with the garlic, vegetable broth, and enough water to cover the cauliflower. Cover and cook on low for 6 hours.

2. Drain the liquid and return the cauliflower to the slow cooker. Add the olive oil, yogurt, turmeric, curry, and ginger and use an immersion blender or potato masher to mash.

3. Serve hot.

Per Serving (1 cup): Calories: 94; Total Fat: 5g; Saturated Fat: 1g; Trans Fat: 0g; Polyunsaturated Fat: 1g; Monounsaturated Fat: 3g; Cholesterol: 0mg; Sodium: 140mg; Carbohydrates: 10g; Fiber: 4g; Sugars: 4g; Protein: 4g

SUBSTITUTION TIP: You can make this side dish dairy-free by replacing the yogurt with a plant-based yogurt or milk.

CARAMELIZED ONIONS AND SHALLOTS

Prep time: 10 minutes / Cook time: 10 to 12 hours on low

The deeply tantalizing sweet flavor of caramelized onions is a marvelous way to take dishes from the ordinary to the extraordinary. The problem is that making them the traditional way on the stove top is tedious and time-consuming. Good news: making them in a slow cooker couldn't be easier! Serve with Chickpea Sloppy Joes (page 97) or Tex-Mex Sloppy Joes (page 130).

Serves 8

8 large Vidalia onions
16 shallots
½ cup extra-virgin olive oil
½ teaspoon salt

1. Halve the onions lengthwise and thinly slice into half-moons. Slice the shallots. Add the onions and shallots to a 6-quart slow cooker. Drizzle with the olive oil and sprinkle the salt over the top and toss to evenly coat.

2. Cover and cook on low for 10 hours, stirring once or twice, if desired. Check to see if the onions are juicy (they release a lot of liquid) and golden-brown. At this point you can stop, or for more concentrated onions and a deeper color, continue cooking for another 2 hours with the cover ajar. Check the onions every hour until they reach your desired taste and color.

3. Remove the onions and shallots with a slotted spoon and use immediately or transfer them to airtight refrigerator or freezer containers. They will keep in the refrigerator for up to 1 week or in the freezer for up to 3 months.

Per Serving (½ cup): Calories: 238; Total Fat: 14g; Saturated Fat: 2g; Trans Fat: 0g; Polyunsaturated Fat: 2g; Monounsaturated Fat: 10g; Cholesterol: 0mg; Sodium: 174mg; Carbohydrates: 28g; Fiber: 3g; Sugars: 17g; Protein: 3g

COOKING TIP: Sweet onions, including Vidalia, Walla Walla, and Maui, are best for this recipe. If you can't find sweet onions, add 1 tablespoon brown sugar to the slow cooker along with the olive oil and salt.

MAPLE-PECAN BRUSSELS SPROUTS

Prep time: **10 minutes** / Cook time: **4 to 5 hours on low**

Roasting Brussels sprouts transforms them from bitter to melt-in-your-mouth delicious. Free up your oven by roasting them in your slow cooker and serve them with your favorite entrée.

Serves 6

2 pounds Brussels sprouts, halved (about 6 cups)

2 red onions, sliced

¼ cup pure maple syrup

2 tablespoons apple cider vinegar

1 tablespoon extra-virgin olive oil

1 teaspoon ground cinnamon

½ cup chopped pecans

1. Put the Brussels sprouts and onions in a 6-quart slow cooker.

2. In a small bowl, stir together the maple syrup, vinegar, cinnamon, and olive oil. Pour this mixture over the vegetables and toss to coat. Cover and cook on low for 4 to 5 hours. The Brussels sprouts should be softened but not mushy.

3. Add the pecans and stir to combine.

Per Serving (1 ⅓ cups): Calories: 176; Total Fat: 10g; Saturated Fat: 1g; Trans Fat: 0g; Polyunsaturated Fat: 3g; Monounsaturated Fat: 6g; Cholesterol: 0mg; Sodium: 50mg; Carbohydrates: 21g; Fiber: 5g; Sugars: 12g; Protein: 4g

NUTRITIONAL HIGHLIGHT: Brussels sprouts are a cruciferous vegetable packed with dietary fiber, folic acid, and high amounts of vitamins A and C. Since they are very low in calories, you can include this superfood often in your heart-healthy eating plan.

PERFECT SWEET POTATOES

Prep time: 5 minutes / Cook time: 7 to 8 hours

Packed with vitamins, minerals, and fiber, sweet potatoes can be incorporated into breakfast, lunch, and dinner. Eggs and sweet potatoes? Delicious. Barbecue chicken over sweet potatoes with a bit of avocado? My absolute favorite. Mashed sweet potatoes? Arguably better than traditional mashed taters. Get creative!

Serves 6

6 sweet potatoes,
    washed and dried

1. Loosely ball up 7 or 8 pieces of aluminum foil and place them in the bottom of a 6-quart slow cooker, covering about half the surface area.

2. Prick each sweet potato 6 to 8 times with a fork. Individually wrap each potato in a piece of foil and seal it completely. Place the wrapped sweet potatoes in the slow cooker on top of the balls of foil.

3. Cover and cook on low for 7 to 8 hours. Use tongs to remove the sweet potatoes from the slow cooker. Allow the potatoes to cool slightly, then unwrap from the foil. Serve hot.

Per Serving (1 potato): Calories: 129; Total Fat: 0g; Saturated Fat: 0g; Trans Fat: 0g; Polyunsaturated Fat: 0g; Monounsaturated Fat: 0g; Cholesterol: 0mg; Sodium: 72mg; Carbohydrates: 30g; Fiber: 4g; Sugars: 6g; Protein: 2g

COOKING TIP: Slow cookers are ideal for saving time. If you don't have an hour to wait at dinnertime for a baked sweet potato, you can throw them in the slow cooker in the morning and they'll be ready when you get home.

LOADED BAKED POTATOES

Prep time: 10 minutes / Cook time: 7 to 8 hours on low

Baking potatoes in a slow cooker is a great no-fuss way to prepare them. This recipe for loaded baked potatoes tops them with homemade Creamy Queso Dip (page 21), cubes of heart-healthy creamy avocado, and chopped fresh chives.

Serves 8

8 Russet potatoes

Extra-virgin olive oil
cooking spray

2 cups Creamy Queso
Dip (page 21)

1 avocado, cubed

½ cup chopped chives

1. Lightly spray the potatoes all over with the olive oil cooking spray. Wrap them individually in aluminum foil and place in a 6-quart slow cooker. Cover and cook for 7 to 8 hours.

2. Remove each potato, slice lengthwise (do not cut the potato fully through), and fluff the inside with the tines of a fork. Add ¼ cup of the queso dip, being careful to keep it inside the potato skins. Rewrap the potatoes in the foil and return them to the slow cooker for 30 minutes more, or until the queso is warmed through.

3. Serve topped with the avocado cubes and chopped chives.

Per Serving (1 potato plus ¼ cup queso): Calories: 372; Total Fat: 9g; Saturated Fat: 5g; Trans Fat: 0g; Polyunsaturated Fat: 1g; Monounsaturated Fat: 3g; Cholesterol: 15mg; Sodium: 280mg; Carbohydrates: 60g; Fiber: 10g; Sugars: 3g; Protein: 13g

NUTRITIONAL HIGHLIGHT: Russet potatoes are often demonized when it comes to weight management. However this vegetable is an excellent source of heart-healthy potassium, vitamins C and B6, and fiber. Just keep an eye on portion sizes.

SPICY VEGAN REFRIED BEANS

Prep time: 5 minutes / Cook time: 10 hours on high

Without the fat but with all of the flavor, these refried beans are a staple in my house. Plus, they have about half the sodium found in canned vegetarian refried beans!

Serves 12

4 cups Savory Vegetable Broth (page 24) or low-sodium vegetable broth

4 cups water

3 cups dried pinto beans

1 onion, chopped

2 jalapeño peppers, minced

4 garlic cloves, minced

1 tablespoon chili powder

2 teaspoons ground cumin

1 teaspoon sweet paprika

1 teaspoon salt

½ teaspoon freshly ground black pepper

1. Combine all of the ingredients in a 4- to 6-quart slow cooker. Cover and cook on high for 10 hours.

2. If there is quite a bit of liquid remaining after cooking, use a ladle to remove some, reserving it in a bowl. Using an immersion blender, blend until smooth or to your desired consistency, adding back the reserved liquid as needed.

3. Serve hot, or freeze in 1- or 2-cup portions in airtight containers.

Per Serving (½ cup): Calories: 91; Total Fat: 0g; Saturated Fat: 0g; Trans Fat: 0g; Polyunsaturated Fat: 0g; Monounsaturated Fat: 0g; Cholesterol: 0mg; Sodium: 127mg; Carbohydrates: 16g; Fiber: 4g; Sugars: 1g; Protein: 5g

COOKING TIP: Slow cookers can cook differently, especially when cooking on high for a prolonged period. If your beans require liquid before blending, add ¼ to ⅓ cup water at a time to obtain the desired consistency. Because of the starch found in beans, the beans will thicken up after blending, so don't fret if they seem thin at first.

SPAGHETTI SQUASH

Prep time: 5 minutes / Cook time: 7 to 8 hours on low

Spaghetti squash is super easy to cook in a slow cooker. There's no need to cut it or peel it. Just poke a few holes in the squash, place it in the slow cooker, set to cook, and forget it. By the end of the day you'll have a healthy, low-calorie, low-carb, fiber-rich alternative to noodles. Serve the squash with Rustic Marinara Sauce (page 16), Creamy Vegan Alfredo Sauce (page 18), Lentil Bolognese (page 92), or another of your favorite seasonings or sauces.

Serves 4

1 spaghetti squash (choose a size that will fit in your slow cooker)

2 cups water

1. Wash your squash with soap and water, and rinse well. With a skewer or fork, puncture 5 or 6 holes in the squash and place it in the slow cooker. Pour in the water. Cover and cook on low for 7 to 8 hours.

2. Carefully remove the squash to a cutting board and allow it to cool for 15 to 20 minutes. Cut the squash in half, and remove and discard the seeds. Using two forks, scrape out the squash strands and put them in a bowl.

Per Serving (1¼ cups): Calories per cup of squash: 52; Total Fat: 0g; Saturated Fat: 1g; Trans Fat: 0g; Polyunsaturated Fat: 1g; Monounsaturated Fat: 4g; Cholesterol: 0mg; Sodium: 34mg; Carbohydrates: 12g; Fiber: 3g; Sugars: 5g; Protein: 1g

COOKING TIP: You can usually fit 2 small squash or 1 large squash in a 6-quart slow cooker. An average 4-pound squash yields about 5 cups of "spaghetti."

CORN ON THE COB

Prep time: 10 minutes / Cook time: 4 to 5 hours on low

There's nothing better than fresh corn on the cob in the summertime! But boiling corn robs it of most of its flavor. In a slow cooker, you are essentially steaming the corn, which keeps the flavors intact. Serve this corn with Salsa Verde Chicken (page 108).

Serves 8

8 corn ears, husked

1 tablespoon extra-virgin olive oil

1 teaspoon freshly ground
   black pepper

1 teaspoon chili powder

¾ cup water

1 small onion, chopped

2 garlic cloves, minced

Butter (optional)

Fresh cilantro (optional)

1. Lightly brush the corn with the olive oil. Season the ears with the black pepper and chili powder and put them in a 6-quart slow cooker.

2. Add the water along with the onion and garlic. Cover and cook on low for 4 to 5 hours, until the corn is bright yellow.

3. Drain and serve, with butter and fresh cilantro, if desired.

Per Serving (1 ear plus 2 tablespoons onion-garlic mixture): Calories: 95; Total Fat: 3g; Saturated Fat: 0g; Trans Fat: 0g; Polyunsaturated Fat: 0g; Monounsaturated Fat: 2g; Cholesterol: 0mg; Sodium: 17mg; Carbohydrates: 19g; Fiber: 3g; Sugars: 3g; Protein: 3g

COOKING TIP: You can tweak the seasonings and use whatever you have on hand. Try fresh sprigs of thyme or rosemary, or 1 teaspoon each of dried basil or dried mustard.

ROASTED PEPPERS

Prep time: 10 minutes / Cook time: 5 to 6 hours on low

Roasted peppers add so much flavor to pasta dishes, grilled meats, and grain dishes. They are also a delicious condiment on sandwiches. And while you can buy jarred roasted peppers, they are usually very salty and expensive. The best part of this slow cooker version is that the bell pepper skin comes off easily after cooking.

Serves 8

Nonstick cooking spray

2 medium yellow bell peppers, halved

2 medium green bell peppers, halved

4 medium red bell peppers, halved

1 large onion, thinly sliced

1 tablespoon extra-virgin olive oil

2 teaspoons dried basil

¼ teaspoon salt

1. Spray the inside of a 6-quart slow cooker with the cooking spray. Add the peppers, onion, olive oil, basil, and salt. Cover and cook on low for 5 to 6 hours.

2. Turn off the slow cooker and remove the lid. Allow the peppers to cool. Grasp a pepper skin at an edge and gently tug to remove it in one piece. If it doesn't come off easily, use a paring knife. Repeat with remaining peppers.

3. Serve immediately with your favorite entrée or store the peppers in an airtight container in the refrigerator for up to 4 days.

Per Serving (⅔ cup): Calories: 70; Total Fat: 2g; Saturated Fat: 0g; Trans Fat: 0g; Polyunsaturated Fat: 1g; Monounsaturated Fat: 1g; Cholesterol: 0mg; Sodium: 77mg; Carbohydrates: 13g; Fiber: 2g; Sugars: 1g; Protein: 2g

VARIATION TIP: This recipe includes an onion for additional flavor, but you can omit it if you have one or simply don't like onions. You can also vary the seasonings and omit the salt, if desired.

RATATOUILLE

Prep time: 10 minutes / Cook time: 7 to 8 hours on low

Slow cookers are perfect for making vegetables meltingly tender with minimal prep or active cooking time. This colorful dish is easy to customize, a type of "kitchen sink" recipe in which you can use up whatever veggies you have on hand. Serve this delicious French classic with your favorite grilled fish or meats.

Serves 8

2 large onions, halved and sliced

1 large eggplant, peeled and
   cut into 2-inch cubes

2 medium zucchini, sliced

2 yellow summer squash, sliced

2 bell peppers (any color),
   cut into strips

4 garlic cloves, minced

2 large tomatoes, cut
   into wedges

2 portobello mushrooms, gills
   and stem removed, sliced

2 teaspoons herbes de
   Provence, divided

2 tablespoons extra-virgin
   olive oil, divided

1 (6-ounce) can tomato
   paste, divided

⅛ teaspoon sugar (optional)

1. Layer half of the onions, eggplant, zucchini, squash, peppers, garlic, tomatoes, and mushrooms, in this order, in the bottom of a 6-quart slow cooker. Sprinkle with 1 teaspoon herbes de Provence and 1 tablespoon olive oil. Dot with half the tomato paste and a sprinkle of the sugar (if using). Repeat the layering process. Cover and cook on low for 7 to 8 hours.

2. Serve hot, with a sprinkle of Parmesan cheese, if desired, on a baguette, over pasta or pizza, or with your favorite entrée.

Per Serving (1¼ cups): Calories: 122; Total Fat: 4g; Saturated Fat: 0g; Trans Fat: 0g; Polyunsaturated Fat: 1g; Monounsaturated Fat: 3g; Cholesterol: 0mg; Sodium: 206mg; Carbohydrates: 21g; Fiber: 5g; Sugars: 8g; Protein: 4g

COOKING TIP: This recipe freezes well. Make a big batch and store it in freezer-safe containers for up to 6 weeks for later use in your favorite recipes.

ROSEMARY-MAPLE BEETS

Prep time: 5 minutes / Cook time: 6 to 8 hours on low

If you are used to eating canned or plain boiled beets, then you will be amazed at how absolutely delicious these slow-roasted beets are. Feel free to switch up the herbs and spices for your favorites.

Serves 6

Nonstick cooking spray

24 baby beets, whole, scrubbed and peeled (or 12 large, quartered)

¼ cup pure maple syrup

¼ cup balsamic vinegar

2 tablespoons extra-virgin olive oil

4 garlic cloves, minced

2 shallots, minced

1 tablespoon minced fresh rosemary, plus additional for garnish

1 teaspoon dried rosemary

1. Spray the inside of a 4- or 6-quart slow cooker with the cooking spray. Place the beets in the slow cooker.

2. In a small bowl, whisk together the maple syrup, vinegar, olive oil, garlic, shallots, fresh rosemary, and dried rosemary.

3. Cover and cook on low for 7 to 8 hours, until the beets are tender. Remove the beets and slice. Serve, garnished with additional rosemary leaves, if desired.

Per Serving (1½ cups): Calories: 154; Total Fat: 5g; Saturated Fat: 1g; Trans Fat: 0g; Polyunsaturated Fat: 1g; Monounsaturated Fat: 3g; Cholesterol: 0mg; Sodium: 124mg; Carbohydrates: 27g; Fiber: 4g; Sugars: 20g; Protein: 3g

COOKING TIP: You can freeze roasted beets for up to 8 months—simply pack them into heavy-duty freezer bags. If the beets are large, slice them first before freezing.

FALL-SPICED APPLESAUCE

Prep time: 20 minutes / Cook time: 4 hours on high or 8 hours on low

Fall spices turn ordinary applesauce into a warm, comforting favorite. After seeing how simple it is to make homemade applesauce, this is sure to be a staple in your kitchen.

Serves 8

5 pounds apples (about 10 large), peeled, cored, and quartered

Juice of 1 lemon

2 teaspoons ground cinnamon

½ teaspoon ground nutmeg

¼ teaspoon ground cloves

¼ teaspoon ground ginger

1. Combine all the ingredients in a 4- or 6-quart slow cooker. Cover and cook on high for 4 hours or low for 8 hours.

2. Mash contents to your desired consistency using a potato masher or a slotted spoon.

3. Serve warm, or refrigerate for up to 5 days.

Per Serving (⅔ cup): Calories: 140; Total Fat: 0g; Saturated Fat: 0g; Trans Fat: 0g; Polyunsaturated Fat: 0g; Monounsaturated Fat: 0g; Cholesterol: 0g; Sodium: 0mg; Carbohydrates: 38g; Fiber: 4g; Sugars: 29g; Protein: 1g

NUTRITIONAL HIGHLIGHT: Notice there's no sugar in this recipe. Slow cooking enhances the natural sweetness of fruit. There's no need for the added sugar found in many store-bought applesauce varieties.

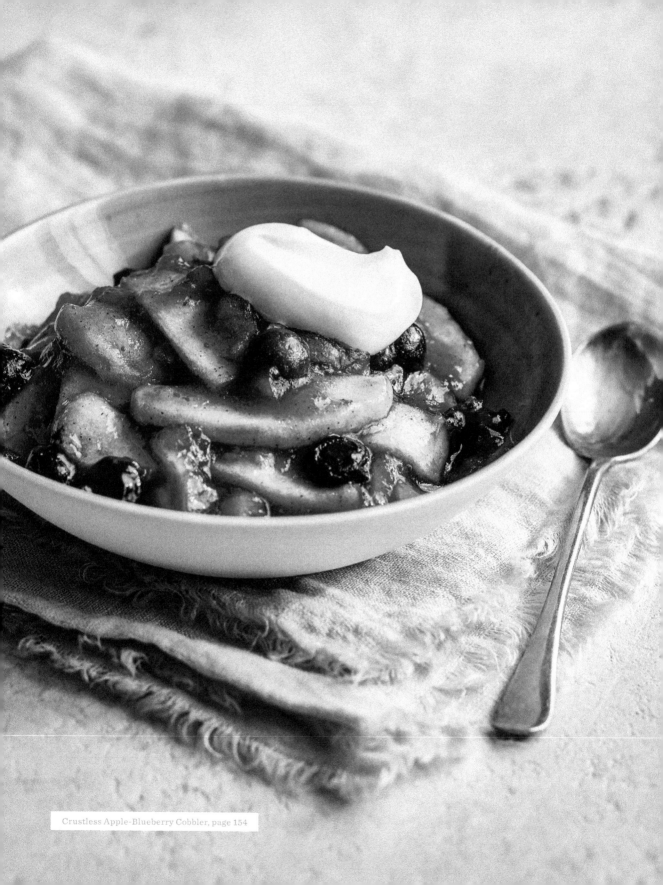

Crustless Apple-Blueberry Cobbler, page 154

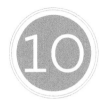

Desserts

CRUSTLESS APPLE-BLUEBERRY COBBLER

Prep time: 15 minutes / Cook time: 2½ to 3 hours on high or 5 to 6 hours on low

The slow cooker is a great tool to use to make desserts, which is something many people don't know. In this dessert, the dried blueberries plump up with the juices from the apples and the cornstarch thickens the whole thing into a masterpiece.

Serves 6

½ cup sugar

2 tablespoons cornstarch

½ teaspoon ground cinnamon

3½ pounds apples (about 8 large) peeled, cored, and cut into ¼-inch slices

1¼ cups dried blueberries

1½ cups low-fat vanilla Greek yogurt

1. In a 4- or 6-quart slow cooker, combine the sugar, cornstarch, and cinnamon. Add the apples and blueberries and mix well to coat.

2. Cover and cook on high for 2½ to 3 hours or low for 5 to 6 hours.

3. Serve hot with ¼ cup yogurt on top of each serving.

Per Serving (¾ cup cobbler with ¼ cup yogurt): Calories: 400; Total Fat: 4g; Saturated Fat: 2g; Trans Fat: 0g; Polyunsaturated Fat: 1g; Monounsaturated Fat: 1g; Cholesterol: 11mg; Sodium: 50mg; Carbohydrates: 92g; Fiber: 8g; Sugars: 78g; Protein: 4g

NUTRITIONAL HIGHLIGHT: Ditch the crust or crumble from traditional cobbler, cutting out loads of fat, calories, and sodium. Instead, showcase the flavor of the fruit. My husband absolutely loves this dessert.

APRICOT-GINGER BROWN RICE PUDDING

Prep time: 10 minutes / Cook time: 5 to 6 hours on low

Slow cooker brown rice pudding is simple to make and a delicious fiber-rich dessert that you can feel good about eating. Dried apricots lend their natural sweetness to this recipe so you need less added sugar. This pudding is also easy to customize with your favorite spices, dried fruits, and nuts.

Serves 6

3½ cups low-fat or fat-free milk, or plant-based milk

⅔ cup brown rice

⅔ cup finely chopped unsweetened dried apricots

¼ cup honey

1 teaspoon ground ginger

1 teaspoon pure vanilla extract

1. Combine all the ingredients to a 6-quart slow cooker. Cover and cook on low for 5 to 6 hours, until the rice is cooked and the pudding is thick. If the pudding is too thick, stir in additional milk; if it is too thin, continue cooking until your desired consistency is reached.

2. The pudding can be served hot, warm, or chilled. Garnish with a dollop of Apple Butter (page 22) or a sprinkle of sliced almonds, if desired.

Per Serving (¾ cup): Calories: 256; Total Fat: 2g; Saturated Fat: 1g; Trans Fat: 0g; Polyunsaturated Fat: 0g; Monounsaturated Fat: 0g; Cholesterol: 8mg; Sodium: 87mg; Carbohydrates: 53g; Fiber: 2g; Sugars: 25g; Protein: 8g

VARIATION TIP: You can also cook this in light canned coconut milk for a creamier consistency. Just note that doing so will increase the calorie and fat content.

MAPLE WALNUTS

Prep time: 5 minutes / Cook time: 2 to 3 hours on low

Walnuts are loaded with health benefits and are the perfect snack to include in a heart-healthy diet. Although they are calorie-dense, small portions of walnuts are satisfying, especially if slow cooked with a maple glaze. This recipe is lower in sugar than traditional candied walnuts yet even more delicious because the slow-cooking process allows the maple syrup to caramelize.

Makes 4 cups

1 pound shelled walnut halves

¼ cup maple syrup

2 tablespoons extra-virgin olive oil

¼ teaspoon ground cinnamon

1 teaspoon vanilla extract

1. Combine all the ingredients in a slow cooker. Cover and cook on low for 2 to 3 hours, stirring once or twice during cooking to make sure the walnuts remain coated.

2. Spread the nuts across parchment paper to cool.

3. Once completely cooled, store in an airtight container in the refrigerator for 2 to 3 months or in the freezer for up to 6 months.

Per Serving (¼ cup): Calories: 213; Total Fat: 20g; Saturated Fat: 2g; Trans Fat: 0g; Polyunsaturated Fat: 14g; Monounsaturated Fat: 4g; Cholesterol: 0mg; Sodium: 0mg; Carbohydrates: 7g; Fiber: 2g; Sugars: 4g; Protein: 4g

VARIATION TIP: If you don't like walnuts simply replace them with your favorite nut, such as pecans or almonds. You could also add dried cranberries for more of a trail mix–type snack.

CHERRY CHOCOLATE CAKE

Prep time: 10 minutes / Cook time: 2 to 2½ hours on low

Cake in a slow cooker? You bet. This delectable cherry chocolate cake has a decadent fudgy taste, but the use of nutritious ingredients keeps the calories and unhealthy fats in check. Easy to prep with basic pantry ingredients, this cake is too scrumptious to resist.

Serves 12

Nonstick cooking spray

1 cup unsweetened cocoa powder

1 cup oat flour, whole-wheat pastry flour, or all-purpose flour

1 cup unsweetened dried cherries

¼ cup ground flaxseed

2 teaspoons baking powder

¼ teaspoon salt

2 tablespoons extra-virgin olive oil

1 large egg

2 large egg whites

1 tablespoon vanilla extract

½ cup granulated sugar

½ cup nonfat vanilla Greek yogurt

¾ cup low-fat or fat-free milk, or plant-based milk, divided

1. Lightly coat the inside of a 6-quart slow cooker with the cooking spray.

2. In a medium bowl, whisk together the cocoa powder, flour, dried cherries, flaxseed, baking powder, and salt.

3. In a separate medium bowl, whisk together the oil, egg, egg whites, and vanilla. Add in the sugar, yogurt, and ¼ cup of milk, mixing thoroughly until no lumps remain. Add the flour mixture and remaining ½ cup of milk, stirring until just combined and incorporated.

4. Spread the batter in the slow cooker. Cover and cook on low for 2 to 2½ hours, or until the center no longer looks moist and feels barely firm to the touch. Remove the lid, turn off the slow cooker, and cool the cake in the ceramic bowl for 15 to 20 minutes before carefully turning it out onto a wire rack to cool completely.

5. Cut into 12 slices and enjoy.

Per Serving (1 slice): Calories: 173; Total Fat: 4g; Saturated Fat: 1g; Trans Fat: 0g; Polyunsaturated Fat: 1g; Monounsaturated Fat: 2g; Cholesterol: 16mg; Sodium: 162mg; Carbohydrates: 31g; Fiber: 5g; Sugars: 16g; Protein: 6g

NUTRITIONAL HIGHLIGHT: Cocoa is an excellent source of heart-healthy antioxidants and plant phytochemicals. A good source of minerals, the flavonoids in cocoa have been shown to have a positive effect on blood pressure.

SPICED BAKED APPLES

Prep time: 15 minutes / Cook time: 4 to 5 hours on low

Baked apples are a healthy, nutritious, and satisfyingly delicious dessert. With minimal prep and just a handful of pantry staples, you can have a fiber- and nutrient-rich dessert in just a few no-fuss hours that the whole family is sure to love.

Serves 6

6 apples

1 cup rolled oats

⅓ cup chopped almonds

2 tablespoons brown sugar

2 teaspoons pumpkin pie spice

½ cup apple juice

2 tablespoons extra-virgin
   olive oil

1. Core the apples using an apple corer or sharp knife. Chop off the top of the apple along with its stem so that the top of the apple is even.

2. In a medium bowl, combine the oats, almonds, brown sugar, and pumpkin pie spice.

3. Stuff the apple cavities with the oat mixture, pressing the mixture down firmly to pack it in. Top off the apples with any remaining oat mixture.

4. Pour the apple juice into a 6-quart slow cooker and carefully add the apples so they are standing upright. Drizzle the apples with the olive oil. Cover and cook on low for 4 to 5 hours, until the apples are tender.

5. Remove the apples from the slow cooker and allow to cool for 5 to 10 minutes before serving.

Per Serving (1 apple with toppings): Calories: 240; Total Fat: 8g; Saturated Fat: 1g; Trans Fat: 0g; Polyunsaturated Fat: 2g; Monounsaturated Fat: 6g; Cholesterol: 0mg; Sodium: 4mg; Carbohydrates: 42g; Fiber: 7g; Sugars: 24g; Protein: 3g

NUTRITIONAL HIGHLIGHT: Apples contain a type of fiber called pectin, which is especially effective for lowering blood cholesterol levels. Most of the fiber in apples is in the skin so wash the apples thoroughly before using and leave the peels on.

DAIRY-FREE • NUT-FREE • VEGETARIAN

VANILLA PEAR CRISP

Prep time: 10 minutes / Cook time: 4 to 5 hours on low

This slow cooker vanilla pear crisp is packed with the delicious flavors of figs, apple, vanilla, nutmeg, and cinnamon. With its contrast of soft-cooked fruit and crunchy oat and nut topping, this healthy dessert pairs nicely with a cup of hot cider.

Serves 6

5 pears, chopped (peeling is optional)

1 apple, chopped (peeling is optional)

½ cup finely chopped dried figs

⅓ cup loosely packed brown sugar

2 teaspoons ground cinnamon

2 teaspoons vanilla extract

1 teaspoon ground nutmeg

½ cup whole-wheat flour, divided

1 cup old-fashioned oats

¼ cup honey

2 tablespoons coconut oil

1. Put the pears, apple, and figs in a 6-quart slow cooker.

2. In a small bowl, combine the brown sugar, cinnamon, vanilla, nutmeg, and ¼ cup of flour. Pour this over the fruit and stir to combine.

3. In the same small bowl, combine the oats, remaining ¼ cup of flour, honey, and coconut oil. Spread this mixture on top of the fruit.

4. Cover and cook on low for 4 to 5 hours, until the fruit is soft.

5. Serve warm.

Per Serving (1⅓ cups): Calories: 305; Total Fat: 6g; Saturated Fat: 4g; Trans Fat: 0g; Polyunsaturated Fat: 1g; Monounsaturated Fat: 1g; Cholesterol: 0mg; Sodium: 4mg; Carbohydrates: 64g; Fiber: 8g; Sugars: 39g; Protein: 4g

SUBSTITUTION TIP: You can make this gluten-free by replacing the whole-wheat flour with coconut flour or almond flour.

MOLASSES-PECAN WHEAT BERRY PUDDING

Prep time: 5 minutes / Cook time: 6 to 8 hours on low

This slow cooker wheat berry pudding is chewy, sweet, spicy, and just plain delicious. Full of fiber, vitamins, and minerals, the molasses gives this nutritious dessert an extra layer of rich flavor. And it's topped with chopped pecans for some heart-healthy fats.

Serves 6

Nonstick cooking spray

1 cup wheat berries

1 ripe banana, mashed

1 tablespoon orange zest

1 teaspoon vanilla extract

1 teaspoon ground cinnamon

½ teaspoon ground nutmeg

1 (2-inch) piece ginger, minced

4 cups low-fat or nonfat milk, or plant-based milk

¼ cup molasses

½ cup chopped pecans

1. Spray the inside of a 6-quart slow cooker with the cooking spray. Add the wheat berries, banana, orange zest, vanilla, cinnamon, nutmeg, and ginger and stir to combine.

2. Pour in the milk and stir well to combine. Cover and cook on low for 6 to 8 hours.

3. Stir in the molasses. Divide the pudding among 6 bowls and garnish with the pecans before serving.

Per Serving (⅔ cup): Calories: 294; Total Fat: 9g; Saturated Fat: 2g; Trans Fat: 0g; Polyunsaturated Fat: 2g; Monounsaturated Fat: 4g; Cholesterol: 10mg; Sodium: 98mg; Carbohydrates: 44g; Fiber: 5g; Sugars: 18g; Protein: 11g

COOKING TIP: For a creamier result, replace ½ cup of milk with ½ cup canned light coconut milk. Just note that doing so will change the nutrition facts.

PUMPKIN PIE OATS

Prep time: 5 minutes / Cook time: 8 to 9 hours

Hearty and packed with fiber, this nutritious twist on a classic fall favorite will have the most heavenly pumpkin pie scents wafting through your house. Serve sprinkled with a tablespoon of ground flaxseed for a dose of heart-healthy omega-3 fatty acids!

Serves 7

2 cups uncooked steel-cut oats

8 cups unsweetened almond milk

1 (15-ounce) can pumpkin purée

1½ tablespoons
   pumpkin pie spice

1½ teaspoons ground cinnamon

⅓ cup brown sugar

1 cup unsalted pecans, chopped

1. Combine the oats, almond milk, pumpkin purée, pumpkin pie spice, cinnamon, and brown sugar in a 4- to 6-quart slow cooker and mix well.

2. Cover with a lid and cook on low for 8 to 9 hours. Stir well and serve warm, topped with pecans.

Per Serving (1½ cups): Calories: 395; Total Fat: 18g; Saturated Fat: 2g; Trans Fat: 0g; Polyunsaturated Fat: 4g; Monounsaturated Fat: 9g; Cholesterol: 0mg; Sodium: 181mg; Carbohydrates: 58g; Fiber: 12g; Sugars: 15g; Protein: 12g

COOKING TIP: Depending on your slow cooker, your oats may still be slightly soupy. They will quickly thicken as they cool. Reheat with a splash of milk in the microwave for 2 to 3 minutes, mixing halfway through.

Measurement & Conversion Tables

VOLUME EQUIVALENTS (LIQUID)

Standard	US Standard (ounces)	Metric (approximate)
2 tablespoons	1 fl. oz.	30 mL
¼ cup	2 fl. oz.	60 mL
½ cup	4 fl. oz.	120 mL
1 cup	8 fl. oz.	240 mL
1 ½ cups	12 fl. oz.	355 mL
2 cups or 1 pint	16 fl. oz.	475 mL
4 cups or 1 quart	32 fl. oz.	1 L
1 gallon	128 fl. oz.	4 L

OVEN TEMPERATURES

Fahrenheit (F)	Celsius (C) (approximate)
250° F	120° C
300° F	150° C
325° F	165° C
350° F	180° C
375° F	190° C
400° F	200° C
425° F	220° C
450° F	230° C

VOLUME EQUIVALENTS (DRY)

Standard	Metric (approximate)
⅛ teaspoon	0.5 mL
¼ teaspoon	1 mL
½ teaspoon	2 mL
¾ teaspoon	4 mL
1 teaspoon	5 mL
1 tablespoon	15 mL
¼ cup	59 mL
⅓ cup	79 mL
½ cup	118 mL
⅔ cup	156 mL
¾ cup	177 mL
1 cup	235 mL
2 cups or 1 pint	475 mL
3 cups	700 mL
4 cups or 1 quart	1 L

WEIGHT EQUIVALENTS

Standard	Metric (approximate)
½ ounce	15 g
1 ounce	30 g
2 ounces	60 g
4 ounces	115 g
8 ounces	225 g
12 ounces	340 g
16 ounces or 1 pound	455 g

The Dirty Dozen™ & the Clean Fifteen™

The Environmental Working Group (EWG) is a nonprofit, nonpartisan organization dedicated to protecting human health and the environment. Its mission is to empower people to live healthier lives in a healthier environment. This organization publishes an annual list of the twelve kinds of produce, in sequence, that have the highest amount of pesticide residue—the Dirty Dozen™—as well as a list of the fifteen kinds of produce that have the least amount of pesticide residue—the Clean Fifteen™.

The Dirty Dozen™

The 2016 Dirty Dozen™ includes the following produce. These are considered among the year's most important produce to buy organic:

Strawberries
Apples
Nectarines
Peaches
Celery
Grapes
Cherries
Spinach
Tomatoes
Bell peppers
Cherry tomatoes
Cucumbers
Kale/collard greens*
Hot peppers*

*The Dirty Dozen™ list contains two additional items—kale/collard greens and hot peppers—because they tend to contain trace levels of highly hazardous pesticides.

The Clean Fifteen™

The least critical to buy organically are the Clean Fifteen™ list. The following are on the 2016 list:

Avocados
Corn**
Pineapples
Cabbage
Sweet peas
Onions
Asparagus
Mangos
Papayas
Kiwi
Eggplant
Honeydew
Grapefruit
Cantaloupe
Cauliflower

** Some of the sweet corn sold in the United States are made from genetically engineered (GE) seedstock. Buy organic varieties of these crops to avoid GE produce.

References

Centers for Disease Control and Prevention. "Heart Disease Fact Sheet." Accessed February 10, 2017. www.cdc.gov/dhdsp/data_statistics/fact_sheets/fs_heart_disease.htm.

Office of Disease Prevention and Health Promotion. "Dietary Guidelines 2015–2020." Accessed February 26, 2018. https://health.gov/dietaryguidelines/2015/guidelines/chapter-1/a-closer-look-inside-healthy-eating-patterns/.

Recipe Index

Index

Acknowledgments

It is with thanks from family, friends, and coworkers that I credit my forever growing passion for nutrition, cooking, and personal impact. I continue to be amazed at all the opportunities that life throws my way and for all of the people in my tribe who rally to support each and every move. Thank you for reading, for cooking, and for always letting my creativity run wild.

About the Author

NICOLE R. MORRISSEY is a Registered Dietician, Certified Diabetes Educator, and cookbook author. She is also the blogger behind Prevention RD, where she hopes to inspire, teach, and keep her readers up to date with the latest developments in nutrition. She has written two other books, *Prevention RD's Everyday Healthy Cooking* and *Prevention RD's Cooking and Baking with Almond Flour*. Nicole lives in southwest Michigan with her husband, two daughters, and English bulldogs. Learn more at https://preventionrd.com.

CPSIA information can be obtained
at www.ICGtesting.com
Printed in the USA
LVHW051412291118
598334LV00003B/3